D0472637

PENGUIN HANDBOOKS

THE INJURED RUNNER'S TRAINING HANDBOOK

Bob Glover is founder and president of Robert H. Glover and Associates, Inc., a fitness consulting firm. He is marketing director and chairman of the Board of Advisors for New York City's prestigious fitness and dining center, the Atrium Club; director of educational programs for the 25,000-member New York Road Runners Club; advisory board member of the 35,000-member American Running & Fitness Association; and fitness director of the Great Wall Run, an educational runners' tour of China. He is also founder and coach of several running teams, including the Achilles Track Club (a club for the physically disabled) and Atalanta (an elite women's team that has won several national championships in both the open and masters categories, has won the New York Marathon four times, and won the Avon International Marathon five times). Glover has more than fifteen years' experience coaching runners of all levels, but he achieves his greatest satisfaction from helping the back-of-the-pack male and female runners increase their enjoyment of the sport. Over 50,000 of these athletes have participated in his classes, and thousands more have followed the training programs in his books.

Dr. Murray Weisenfeld has been a podiatrist in New York City for over thirty years. In his private practice he treats hundreds of athletes from many sports, including runners, dancers, baseball players, and tennis players. Dr. Weisenfeld is a member of the advisory board for the Atrium Club and *New Body* magazine and is a Fellow of the Academy of Sports Podiatry. His first book, *The Runner's Repair Manual*, has been successful around the world.

Also by Bob Glover

The Runner's Handbook: The Classic Fitness Guide for Beginning and Intermediate Runners
by Bob Glover and Jack Shepherd

The Runner's Handbook Training Diary
by Bob Glover and Jack Shepherd

The Competitive Runner's Handbook: The Complete Training Program for All Distance Running
by Bob Glover and Pete Schuder

Also by Dr. Murray Weisenfeld, Podiatrist

The Runner's Repair Manual: A Complete Program for Diagnosing and Treating Your Foot, Leg, and Back Problems
by Dr. Murray Weisenfeld and Barbara Burr

THE INJURED RUNNER'S TRAINING HANDBOOK

The Coach's and Doctor's Guide for Preventing, Running Through, and Coming Back from Injury

BOB GLOVER *and* MURRAY WEISENFELD, D.P.M.

PENGUIN BOOKS

PENGUIN BOOKS
Viking Penguin Inc., 40 West 23rd Street,
New York, New York 10010, U.S.A.
Penguin Books Ltd, Harmondsworth,
Middlesex, England
Penguin Books Australia Ltd, Ringwood,
Victoria, Australia
Penguin Books Canada Limited, 2801 John Street,
Markham, Ontario, Canada L3R 1B4
Penguin Books (N.Z.) Ltd, 182–190 Wairau Road,
Auckland 10, New Zealand

First published in Penguin Books 1985

Published simultaneously in Canada

LIBRARY OF CONGRESS CATALOGING IN PUBLICATION DATA
Glover, Bob.
   The injured runner's training handbook.
   Includes index.
   1. Running—Training.   2. Running—Accidents and
injuries.   I. Weisenfeld, Murray F.   II. Title.
GV1061.5.G545   1985   796.4'26   84-26541
ISBN 0 14 046.641 X

Printed in the United States of America by
R. R. Donnelley and Sons Company, Harrisonburg, Virginia
Set in Electra

DEDICATION

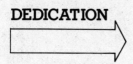

To Dr. Richard O. Schuster, pioneer of sports medicine
for runners

ACKNOWLEDGMENTS We have a combined experience of over sixty years in the running world. During these years we have had the good fortune to have coached or treated thousands of fine people. We have shared in their joys and frustrations as they have struggled through injuries and returned to the running paths. One always learns more from his athletes and patients than he teaches. In this regard, we are deeply indebted to all those runners who have sought our counsel and made us wiser men.

Bob Glover especially wishes to thank the elite runners of his women's team, Atalanta—five-time Avon International Marathon Club Champions—who patiently (usually) experimented with his theories on alternative training. He is particularly grateful to the women who are used as models in this book: Cindi Girard, Angella Hearn, Robin Ladas, Paula Morrell, Patty Lee Parmalee, and Kass Young. Glover reserves special praise once again for Jack Shepherd, who coauthored *The Runner's Handbook*, helped write *The Competitive Runner's Handbook*, and contributed to this work.

We also thank biker-runners Lou Kwiker, Vince McDonald, and Eric Ryan and swimmer-runner John Bell for their advice, and thank Richard Traum, the veteran one-legged marathoner and president of the Achilles Track Club (for the physically disabled). A special thanks to John Brodhead, triathlon athlete and director of the Craftsbury (Vermont) Sports Camp, for reviewing the alternative training chapters.

Bob Glover also thanks the various doctors, in addition to Dr. Weisenfeld, who have treated his injuries and illnesses over the years and patiently answered his many questions about how to keep his runners on the road: Dr. Milton Brothers, Dr. Edward Colt, Dr. Fred Grabo, Dr. Hans Kraus, Dr. Norbert Sander, Dr. Richard Schuster, and Dr. George Sheehan.

Dr. Weisenfeld is grateful to his professional colleagues Dr. Seymour (Mac) Goldstein, chiropractor; Dr. Stanley Roman, osteopath; Dr. Richard Schuster, podiatrist; Dr. Hans Kraus, specialist in physical medicine; and orthopedists Dr. Fisk Warren, Dr. James Parkes, and Dr. William Hamilton.

In addition, the New York City physical therapist and Atrium Club consultant Robert Kropf deserves special thanks for his rehabilitation work with the Atalanta athletes and his extensive review of and valued input for this book.

We both thank our wives, Virginia Glover and Shirley Weisenfeld, and our children, Christopher Glover, Lori Weisenfeld, Irv Weisenfeld, Harry Weisenfeld, and Janet Skolnik, for their lifelong support of our careers and their enduring love.

PREFACE

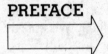

The role of a coach is to train an athlete to a high level of fitness and to push him or her to perform well in competition. Often the coach and the athlete lose sight of the fact that overtraining can lead to injury and loss of fitness. Coaches and athletes need to be as aware of the causes and warning signs of injury as they are knowledgeable about sound training practices. As every runner knows, breakdown will invariably occur. When it does, the coach and athlete need to work together with the sports-medicine professional to keep the runner on the road to fitness.

In treating a runner's injury, the doctor often has goals different from those of the athlete and the coach. The doctor generally views an injury with a conservative eye and prescribes a traditional remedy, such as time off from training. However, with the increased popularity of jogging and competitive running in the 1970s and 1980s, the medical profession has been forced to recognize that runners desperately want to keep running despite nagging injury and if forced to stop training want to return as quickly as possible. Thus, the specialty of sports medicine has grown tremendously in response to the running boom, and doctors have learned ways to help runners not only treat injuries and prevent reoccurrence, but continue running while minimizing further injury. Coaches have learned to adjust training methods and doctors to adjust injury treatment in order to provide the injured runner with a safe, yet progressive return to the roads and good health.

Bob Glover has coached over 50,000 men, women, and children and has been a competitive runner for over twenty years. He has learned from experience about every type of injury and about how to continue training when injured. Glover has become a better coach through his relationships with Dr. Murray Weisenfeld, who has treated thousands of athletes over the last thirty years, and Dr. Richard Schuster. They and others in sports medicine have taught him how to adjust a training program to meet the needs of the injured runner safely. Dr. Weisenfeld, meanwhile, has benefited from his exposure to Bob Glover and other coaches. By becoming more aware of a runner's training methods, errors, and competitive psychology, a doctor can more competently assist an injured athlete. Over the years Glover and Weisenfeld have worked closely with hundreds of runners from Glover's running classes and his elite women's team, Atalanta. They have shared ideas about how to treat an injury properly and how to adjust the runner's training program. From these experiences comes the training and recovery program in this book.

Although the coach and doctor can learn a great deal from each other that can assist an injured runner, one important point should always be stressed: A coach shouldn't doctor and a doctor shouldn't coach. The goal of this book—the first of its kind—is to provide you with both a coach's and a doctor's guide to preventing, training through, and coming back from injury. We hope that the collaborative effort will make you an injury-free, productive runner.

CONTENTS

ACKNOWLEDGMENTS   vii

PREFACE   ix

INTRODUCTION: KEEPING THE RUNNER ON THE ROAD TO FITNESS AND BETTER RACE TIMES   xiii

PART I: PREVENTION OF INJURIES   1

   1. WHO AND WHAT GETS INJURED   3

   2. PREVENTING INJURIES   8

PART II: TRAINING THROUGH AND COMING BACK FROM INJURY   27

   3. PSYCHOLOGICAL ASPECTS OF INJURY   29

   4. RUNNING THROUGH AN INJURY   34

   5. COMING BACK FROM A LAYOFF   40

PART III: THE AFTERMARATHON   51

   6. PREVENTING INJURY AFTER RUNNING THE MARATHON   53

PART IV: ALTERNATIVE TRAINING   65

   7. HOW TO CHOOSE AND USE ALTERNATIVE AEROBIC TRAINING   67

   8. BIKING   79

   9. SWIMMING   90

  10. WALKING   102

  11. RACE WALKING   106

  12. CROSS-COUNTRY SKIING   110

PART V: MANAGEMENT OF INJURY   117

  13. TREATMENT OPTIONS   119

  14. SPECIAL AIDS: INSOLES, HEEL LIFTS, TAPING, AND ORTHOTICS   139

  15. DRUGS AND RUNNING   153

  16. SPECIFIC TREATMENTS FOR COMMON RUNNING INJURIES   159

  17. SPECIAL EXERCISES FOR SPECIFIC INJURIES   178

INDEX   197

INTRODUCTION: KEEPING THE RUNNER ON THE ROAD TO FITNESS AND BETTER RACE TIMES

An estimated 20 million American adults run on a regular basis. Of these, at least one-third are likely to seek medical attention for running-related injuries each year. The more serious the runner, and the more he or she abuses the body with high mileage, the higher the chance of injury. Some studies show that as many as 75 percent of runners who train over 50 miles per week get injured at least once a year. According to Dr. Lyle Micheli, director of the division of sports medicine at Children's Hospital Medical Center in Boston, "Running is the most dangerous sport in the United States in terms of the numbers of injuries we are seeing." He adds that most often these injuries are caused by training errors.

Fortunately, there are very few permanent injuries caused by running. Long Beach, California, podiatrist John Pagliano and orthopedist Douglas Jackson delivered the results of a six-year study of 3,000 injured runners at the 1984 Annual Meeting of the American College of Sports Medicine. They stated: "Distance running is associated with a low incidence of disabling injuries. Although running places a heavy load on the musculoskeletal system, particularly the back and lower extremities, very few of the injuries sustained will preclude the runner's return to his or her desired mileage and training program."

Health is something you pass on your way to being a competitive runner. Competitive running contributes little to health and fitness. In truth, it tears one down more than it builds one up. But competitive runners are running for sport, not fitness. Like other athletes, they must learn to accept the inevitability of injury and illness and to minimize its effect on their ability to perform.

It is safe to say that every year of competitive running will find you injured or ill at least a few times. Your best and safest response is to be conservative, hold back, and return cautiously to running. For the competitive runner, there is a fine line between overtraining and undertraining. Too much training can lead to injury and illness, too little may lead to underachievement. You will determine your own outer limits and strive for the injury-free competitive area between. Often this is what makes the difference between winning and losing, or simply reaching the goal of a personal record, at all levels of competition. The key ingredients of success in competitive running are most often thought to be natural talent, hard training, and a strong mental attitude. Improvement for most runners is also closely linked to the ability to stay injury-free. When injury does occur, the successful runner wisely alters his or her training while the injury is being treated. Many runners get into great shape only to become injured or ill and never make it to the starting line. The runner who loses training time again and again will be in worse shape than the conservative and consistent runner.

There is no need to stop training just because of the risks of injury. Accept the fact that it is a part of the sport, but learn how to minimize it. Don't give up in frustration if you develop a nagging injury. Learn how to treat it properly and how to adjust your training to keep in shape while warding it off. This book will serve as your guide to coping with injuries and keeping on the road to fitness and better race times.

Runners must overcome two obstacles: the injuries arising from inactivity, which are discovered when one is getting into shape; and then the injuries of excellence, which sometimes come from running too well. The sedentary man or woman is often faced with a life of illnesses and physical problems: obesity, high blood pressure, tension, weak muscles, a lack of energy. As one begins running, the most common cause of injury is trying to do too much too soon. (The training guidelines in *The Runner's Handbook* safely teach beginners and intermediate-level runners how to achieve fitness and minimize injury.) Once a runner adjusts to 20–30 minutes of running, three to five times a week—the minimal amount for good fitness—he or she seldom gets injured. Indeed, studies show that very few who run 6–9 miles a week need medical attention during a year's time. But, when the runner decides to become a competitor and increase mileage, add speed work, and begin to race, the risk of injury dramatically increases. Again, the most common cause of injury is trying to do too much too soon.

There are other books for runners about how to treat injuries or how to train if you are healthy. But this is the first to explain how an injured runner can maintain his or her training program. Our guidelines for running through and coming back from injury will help you use alternative training to enhance your performance. Our advice will also help you prevent injury. But if you should become ill or injured, this book will help you maintain fitness and put you back on the road again in great shape.

Part I
PREVENTION OF INJURIES

1 WHO AND WHAT GETS INJURED

During the early- to mid-1970s, *Runner's World* surveyed its readers four different times about running injuries. Not surprisingly, some 60 to 70 percent said that they had suffered a running-related injury during the previous year which had limited their training. A 1982 survey of 10,754 runners by La Jolla, California, podiatrist Joe Ellis revealed that 76 percent of them had sustained an injury in their running career which had at some time forced them to discontinue running. Of some 2,500 runners who were surveyed at the 1983 Peachtree 10-kilometer road race in Atlanta, over 35 percent had suffered a musculoskeletal injury within the year that was severe enough for them to cut back seriously on their mileage. Only 10 percent of runners who ran 6–9 miles per week sought medical attention during the year according to the Atlanta survey, compared with 35 percent of those running over 50 miles per week. These statistics back up what Dr. Weisenfeld sees in his practice: As mileage creeps up past 40 miles per week and the body absorbs more pounding, flexibility and muscle balance are affected and the incidence of injuries increases. He and Bob Glover also observe more injuries among runners who tend to overtrain for key races, particularly the marathon, than among those who train more casually for shorter key races. Over 1,000 of the 16,000 runners accepted for the 1984 New York Marathon were forced to cancel because of injury or illness. Greed, trying to get one more good race out of a tired body, is often the cause of injury for experienced competitors. Runners who have just started racing are most often guilty of wanting too much too soon.

The incidence of injuries to women runners is about the same as that for men. As Dr. Leslie S. Matthews of Baltimore's Union Memorial Hospital Sports Medicine Center jokes, "Women are equally entitled to athletic injury. . . . Most injuries women suffer are sports related, not gender related." Common gender-related injuries to women are groin injuries and pelvic fractures, caused by the fact that women have broader pelvises than men. Dr. Weisenfeld treats a variety of injuries to women caused by wearing high-heeled shoes. Common problems include pain in the ball of the foot resulting from the forward thrust of weight and pain in the Achilles tendon and calf created by the prolonged raising of the heel.

Some studies indicate that women may be slightly more prone to injuries than men. In Dr. Ellis's survey 5 percent fewer men than women reported injury, probably because women tend to pronate (turn inward) more than men.

Dr. Richard Schuster noted in *The Runner*: "Although female runners are said to be more prone to injury than their male counterparts, my experience does not bear this out. Women develop more injuries of certain types and fewer of others. This is partly because of their body structure and chemistry . . . women tend to be much more flexible and derive from that measurably greater joint ranges. This reduces the incidence of many injuries caused by lack of flexibility such as muscle pulls and Achilles tendinitis. . . . The average woman has hips that are relatively wide to accommodate childbearing. This causes the upper legs to slant in and come together at the knee. There's a wide range of individual difference in how marked this tendency is—some women have very straight leg bones, others slant so much they become knock-kneed. Not only can the inward slanting of the upper legs decrease running efficiency by causing cross-striding, it can also lead to injury, especially chondromalacia—runner's knee. . . . Women appear to sustain more stress fractures in the lower leg than men. Again, this is because their bones tend to be more curved. Women's bones are also smaller and therefore more susceptible to the force of impact."

Robert Kropf, a physical therapist who specializes in the rehabilitation of runners, believes that many of women's injuries are related to poor strength in the muscles surrounding the hip joint. This lack of strength can be a major contributing factor to injury throughout the entire lower leg. Runners need good strength at the hip to provide a firm base of support. This enables the muscles of the lower leg to work efficiently and injury-free. Without this support, instability will be transmitted down the leg, thereby increasing the likelihood of injury at the knee, ankle, and foot.

As we age, our bodies begin to betray us. We become more brittle and less flexible and gradually lose muscle strength. We recover more slowly from long or hard runs, and require more easy days. The gradual loss of bone mass—especially in women—increases the risk of fractures and retards the healing of bone injuries. Dr. Weisenfeld finds that his older patients are more prone to heel spur formation but generally have fewer injuries than younger runners. Older beginning runners are usually more cautious, and wily veterans of the roads who have experienced a variety of injuries know how to hold injuries off.

Young runners are particularly susceptible to injury where bone union occurs in the soft plates at the heel, and in the tibia (shin) just below the knee. These plates, called apophyses, gradually close with adolescence, but serious damage to them can delay growth. Experts in sports medicine disagree about whether very young athletes who try long-distance running are risking serious injury. Dr. Weisenfeld has found that ten- to twelve-year-olds often develop a separation at the heelbone, usually because they hit too hard on their heels or their shoes lack proper cushioning. Girls aged eleven to fourteen and boys fourteen to sixteen are prone to Osgood-Schlatters disease, which is a separation of the epiphyseal line where the head of the tibia meets the shaft of the tibia. This disease can cause a delay in growth, resulting in a shortened limb and pain below the knee.

Over the last decade, the types of injuries that runners get has changed. In 1980 doctors at the St. Elizabeth's Hospital Sports Medicine Runner's Clinic in Boston conducted a study on 1,000 runners. They looked at the types of injuries reported and compared the results with those of earlier *Runner's World* surveys to see if the injury pattern had changed with increased awareness among runners of physiology and the greater sophistication of sports medicine. Lloyd S. Smith, D.P.M., observed in *Running & Fitness* that knee complaints increased from 25 percent to 30.5 percent, heel spurs and plantar fasciitis increased from 10 to 13.4 percent, and shinsplints and related stress fractures also increased, from 10 to 20.6 percent. Achilles tendinitis decreased from 18 percent to only 6 percent. A study by Dr. John Pagliano and Dr. Douglas Jackson reported in *Runner's World* revealed similar findings: increases in injuries to the knee, shins, and heels, along with a decrease in Achilles tendinitis.

The types of injuries have changed over the years because runners have learned the value of stretching exercises to minimize some injuries, but not how to protect themselves against the kinds of injuries brought on with higher mileage. Improvements in running shoes have decreased some injuries, but increased others. Dr. Weisenfeld reports increases over the years in knee injuries, heel spurs, plantar fasciitis, and stress fractures as well as shinsplints on the inner side of the leg. He feels that these increases are linked to higher mileage and softer-soled shoes. His patients complain less frequently of Achilles tendinitis or shinsplints in the front of the legs. This is probably so because of increased flexibility in both runners and shoes and the use of heel lifts. Injuries to the forefoot have also increased, probably as a result of runners' landing on the balls of their feet as they attempt to go faster in speed work and races.

Of the 1,077 patients in the Pagliano-Jackson survey, 566 reported foot problems, 322 suffered knee injuries, 472 reported injuries to the skeletal system, 275 to the posterior muscular system, and 157 to the anterior muscular system. Thus it seems that runners are most vulnerable in their bones and joints; the antigravity or "pushing" muscles (back), which do most of the work in running, are more prone to injury than the "pulling" muscles (front).

2 PREVENTING INJURIES

An important part of running, especially for the competitive runner, is learning to prevent injuries and illnesses. The runner must accept that "diseases of excellence" are a part of the sport, but try to minimize their effect on his or her training. Injuries seldom occur as a result of accident; most often they seem just to happen for no reason at all.

Most runners' injuries and illnesses have one of four causes: inherited physical weaknesses, improper health practices, environmental influences, and the most frequent cause, training errors. Few running injuries are caused by a single factor or event, such as one particular speed workout or race. Underlying the occurrence of a shinsplint may be several contributing causes, such as poor running form, a biomechanically weak foot, and worn-down running shoes. Running injuries do not occur suddenly. They are caused by a gradual and often predictable overstressing of a susceptible part of the body. Your body will give off warning signals that injury is likely to occur. Thus, two ways to prevent injury are to identify and eliminate the causes and listen to the warning signs.

To identify the reasons you get injured or ill, answer the questions in the injury and illness checklist.

INJURY AND ILLNESS CHECKLIST

These are some of the questions we ask runners who become injured or ill. The goal is to identify the reason or reasons they developed their problems. Often more than one factor is involved. The basic question is: What have you done differently in your running or daily routine that may have caused the injury or illness?

Training Errors
1. Have you made any sudden changes in the quantity or quality of your runs? Have you increased your mileage or speed or added hill work? Are you overtraining—wanting too much too soon?
2. Are you undertrained for the races you're running?
3. Are you racing too frequently?
4. Are you taking time to recover from races and hard workouts?
5. Did you return from recent injury or illness too quickly?
6. Is your running form proper?
7. Do you have good flexibility?
8. Do you warm up and cool down correctly for all runs?
9. Do you overstretch?
10. Are your opposing muscles weak?
11. Have you fallen victim to "marathonitis"?

Inherited Physical Weaknesses
1. Are your feet structurally weak?
2. Are your legs of unequal length?

Improper Health Practices
1. Has your weight changed? Are you overweight or underweight?

2. Is your diet adequate for your training level?
3. Are you taking proper care of your feet?
4. Have you changed any daily habits? Are you driving or sitting more?
5. Have you been doing other sports that might affect your running?
6. Are you under additional stress?
7. Are you getting enough sleep?

Environmental Influences
1. Has running on snow or ice changed your running pattern or form?
2. Have you changed running surfaces, or are you running on uneven or slanted terrain? Are you running hard on downhills with improper form?
3. Have you changed running shoes? Are your running shoes worn down? Have you started to wear racing shoes?

IDENTIFYING AND ELIMINATING THE CAUSES OF INJURY AND ILLNESS

The following summary of causes of injuries and illnesses will help you answer the checklist questions; it also offers some suggestions about how you can eliminate these causes and prevent future injury.

Training Errors
1. *Overtraining—Too Much Mileage, Speed, or Hill Work.*
According to E. C. Frederick, Ph.D., who is the director of research and development for Nike, Inc., the leading cause of overtraining and injury is "Too much too soon. That's almost always the case. It's the athlete's urge to do more, exceeding his or her body's ability to adapt. You hark back to Selye's theory about adaptation. You have a certain capacity to adapt, and once you exceed that, it triggers the symptoms of overtraining, which may be a

protective physiological response to too much stress."

Too much mileage too soon may be the leading cause of injury to all runners. Even if you build up your mileage gradually, beyond a certain point you may be unable to handle more. Dr. Lyle Micheli adds that he sees "a real increase in injuries when people get beyond 50 miles a week in running. It's like a medical barrier. All kinds of problems develop, from tendinitis to irritation of the soles of the feet, to knee problems." We feel the solution may be orthotics, or holding the mileage at a level below that which causes problems until the body is ready to accept more mileage.

Speed work helps you race faster. Unfortunately, it also increases your chance of injury. There is a very fine line between speed work which produces physiological benefits and that which causes injury. With experience, you will develop a feel for what is safe for you and still provides training benefits. Also, sudden changes in the speed of your daily training runs may result in fatigue and injury.

Hill work is a specialized type of speed training. Fast runs uphill place a severe stress on the lower leg and can cause lower-back and hamstring injury. Keep away from hill workouts when your Achilles tendons, shins, or calves are troubling you or when you are recovering from hard races or long runs. Also, beware that sudden changes in the number and quality of hills in your daily runs may cause injury.

2. *Undertraining.* You must have the mileage base and speed training to be prepared for races. Overtraining often causes you to break down before you reach the starting line, but undertraining often causes you to break down before you reach the finish line.

3. *Greed—Racing Too Frequently.* You can stress yourself physically and mentally with too much racing. Select and space your races wisely, and allow yourself to recover before applying the race stress again.

4. *Inadequate Recovery*. The training effect won't take place if you don't allow your body to recover from stress. Follow the hard-easy method of training. You may need additional easy days or even days off following stressful workouts and races. Bob Glover developed a policy of discouraging his top runners from running a step for two days after any race over 10 kilometers. Instead, they bike or swim, to minimize the trauma to their musculoskeletal systems. This aids recovery without increasing the chance of injury.

5. *Returning Too Quickly from Injury and Illness*. Take your time! Allow an injury to heal before running hard or long again, and don't resume training too soon after illness. Relapses are common, causing loss of even more training time. Many serious injuries result from ignoring or favoring a minor injury. According to physical therapist Robert Kropf, "unfortunately many runners don't realize that once you have an injury your body will adjust unconsciously and shift stress away from the point of pain. Any alteration in biomechanics predisposes runners to injury in other areas of that same leg, or, as I have seen, most often injury in the opposite leg. In my practice, I ask runners to alternately lift one leg up and balance on the opposite leg to test balance and weight shifting. In 90 percent of the cases, I see poorer balance capabilities on the injured side and increased weight shifting away from the injury."

According to the survey by Dr. John Pagliano and Dr. Douglas Jackson, 21 percent of runners' problems were recurring injuries or incomplete recoveries from previous problems, while 79 percent were first-time injuries.

6. *Errors in Running Form*. Technique is important for both fast running and healthy running. A pronounced forward lean will result in extra pressure on the lower leg. Leaning backward, "braking," will cause pressure on the back and hamstring muscles. Swaying from side to side and running too "tight" may also cause injury. Overstriding—when your foot hits in front of your center of gravity—makes the surface push your body back, and this stress often causes shinsplints and stress fractures. Running too hard on the heel at footstrike or too high on the ball of the foot may cause injury. When you are concerned about preventing injury, run heel-ball, hitting lightly on the heel. When concerned about improving speed, run ball-heel, but not way up on the toes. If you cross your arms in front of your body as you run, the swaying may cause hip or lower-back pain. Be alert to warning signs of injury.

7. *Poor Flexibility.* Tight or shortened muscles are more easily injured than stretched muscles and cause a variety of biomechanical problems. Stretching both before and after running is essential for the Achilles tendon, the calf and hamstring muscles, and the back and hips. Stretching improves flexibility, and a flexible body is more fluid in motion, more efficient, and able to run faster.

8. *Incorrect Warm-up and Cool-down.* Too many runners warm up and cool down improperly. This can cause more injuries than it prevents. The warm-up should consist of relaxation and limbering and gentle stretching exercises, followed by more detailed stretching. Start your run slowly, and after a mile or two ease into your training pace. After your run, reverse this procedure. Many feel that this is the most effective and safest time to stretch because the muscles are warm. Gradually bring your pulse down by walking and then by doing easy stretches followed by more advanced ones. If you are very fatigued—such as after a long run or hard speed workout or race—do only light stretching and walking. After a workout, do not collapse in a heap: Force yourself to walk, stretch, and recover with a proper cool-down. The cool-down minimizes fatigue and soreness following vigorous activity.

9. *Overstretching.* Overzealous or careless stretching can do more harm than good. Never jerk or bounce when you stretch, and stretch only to the point where you feel a mild pulling sensa-

tion. Do not stretch injured muscles; this will only aggravate the injury and delay healing. Leave the muscle alone until tenderness and swelling disappear, then gradually work to improve its flexibility. If you have a recurring problem such as back pain, don't do any exercise that aggravates it.

10. *Muscle Imbalance.* It is important that muscles be strong and that opposing muscles have a proper balance of strength. The prime contracting or agonist muscles (buttocks, hamstrings, and calf muscles) become overdeveloped and tight with running. Stretching exercises for these muscles coupled with strengthening exercises for the opposing antagonist muscles are essential to restore muscle groups to proper balance. Otherwise, imbalances lead to injury. Strengthening exercises to prevent injuries include those for the abdominal muscles (easing back pain), shin-area muscles (shinsplints), and quadriceps in the thigh (hamstring and knee pain).

11. *Marathonitis.* Too many people are training for and running in marathons before they are properly prepared. Actually, marathons themselves cause few injuries. But overmileage or improper preparation sidelines thousands of runners. Those who get injured during the marathon are mostly undertrained runners or those who ran with injuries against their doctors' advice. An additional complication is that injuries developed or aggravated during the race are most often ignored during the marathon. In a shorter race the runner would probably drop out, but the marathoner feels obligated to suffer, since it is part of the glory. Another problem is coming back to training too soon after a marathon (see Chapter 6).

The majority of veteran marathoners would be better off limiting themselves to one or two marathons a year. One should be the maximum for less experienced racers. Marathons are not easy. They are very challenging. Proper training and preparation are essential.

Inherited Physical Weaknesses

1. *Structurally Weak Feet.* Many runners have biomechanically weak feet. This means that their feet have some basic physical flaw that, aggravated by running, leads to foot, leg, or knee injuries. With weak feet, the force exerted upon footstrike (1,000 times during every mile of running at three to four times the runner's weight) causes an abnormal strain on the supporting tendons, muscles, and fasciae of the feet and legs. Orthotics, either commercially made or custom fitted by a podiatrist, may help runners with this problem (see Chapter 13).

2. *Unequal Leg Length.* If your legs are of different lengths, you may experience pain in your back, knees, or hips. In many cases, unequal leg length causes no injury. When it does, the injury often occurs first on the long leg. Structural shortages may be anywhere in the leg: the upper leg, the lower leg, or below the ankle. Heel lifts or orthotics to balance leg length may help; placed inside the shoe, they should never exceed half an inch. If you experience back, hip, or knee problems, have a sports-medicine expert check for leg-length discrepancy before you spend a lot of money for other treatment. This is one of the most neglected causes of running injuries and one of the easiest to repair.

Improper Health Practices

1. *Body Weight.* Your bone structure, metabolism, and personal preference will dictate what is too little or too much weight for you. Losing weight too rapidly may make you weak and ill; being underweight may have the same effect. Dr. Edward Colt, an endocrinologist at New York City's St. Luke's Hospital, observes that "the lighter you are, within certain limits, the less likely you are to become injured. The limits are set by your own constitution—each individual has an optimum weight below which he or she becomes susceptible to infections." If you are 20

percent or more over your "ideal" weight, you must get your weight down before racing to prevent injury. The runner who is 30 pounds overweight slams the ground with 20 percent more force than normal.

2. *Inadequate Diet.* Eat a balanced diet, and don't fool around with food fads. Proper nutrition is important to everyone's health.

3. *Improper Foot Care.* Wash and dry your feet properly and regularly and use antifungal powder to prevent athlete's foot. Corns, warts, infections, slivers, ingrown toenails, and the like should be taken care of immediately by your podiatrist. Also take care of blisters and calluses promptly and properly (see pages 175–177). Minor foot problems can lead to major discomfort and lost training time, or to injuries caused by favoring these problems.

4. *Daily Habits.* A sudden change in daily habits can cause problems, especially back pain or sciatica. Avoid changes in posture at home or at the office, standing or sitting too much, reaching or lifting. Driving long distances, especially when you are unaccustomed to it, can cause tightened muscles and strains in the back. Use correct form when lifting heavy objects. Sleep on a firm mattress and in the proper position—not on your stomach or back, but on your side in the fetal position. If you experience pain, always look for a change in daily habits as a possible cause.

5. *Other Sports.* When you reach the competitive level of running, you have to decide which other sports you want to participate in and what their benefits and risks might be. Besides the obvious risks of sprains and breaks in such sports as skiing and basketball, you run the risk of injury because muscles that have been tightened by running are not as flexible as they once were, making you less agile and less resistant to injury. If you want to participate in other sports as well as maximize your potential as a runner, be very moderate in your activity. You should do much less of another sport than you can handle in terms of heart and lung conditioning because your muscles will not tell you that you have overdone it until it is too late—a day or two afterward. Also, do not use thick-soled running shoes for change-of-direction sports such as tennis and volleyball—they are made for maximum cushioning for forward motion and using them for anything else will make you susceptible to ankle sprains.

6. *Stress.* "Stress," says Dr. Hans Selye, author of *Stress Without Distress* and *The Stress of Life,* "is essentially the wear and tear in the body caused by life at any one moment." Stress causes physical changes and may cause a variety of medical ills as well, some imagined and some very real, painful, even lethal. Each period of stress, Dr. Selye says, especially from frustrating, unsuccessful struggles, leaves some irreversible chemical scars. When burdened beyond our stress tolerance, we become ill or develop emotional problems, or suffer the physical breakdowns of athletes. Stress takes its physiological toll. Our emotions affect our muscles, and our muscles reflect our emotional problems.

Some runners run with stress, carrying their tensions visibly during a workout. They run with tight muscles, tense and high shoulders, and short, choppy strides. They are too busy to relax, warm up, stretch, and begin running slowly before beating their bodies into the hard, paved road. As a consequence, they often pay the penalty of tight calves and hamstrings, as well as back pain.

In the beginning, when you take up the sport of running, the exercise helps you cope with stress. But after you get into competitive racing, it can become an additional stress, which may overwhelm you. Stress, whether caused by the drive to become a better runner or by external factors, makes you vulnerable to illness and injury.

Injuries often go hand in hand with life transitions, long periods of work overload, or both. Several studies have shown an increased risk of illness, injuries, and accidents among people scoring high on stress checklists associated with changes in life. Dr. Walt Schafer and Dr. John McKenna of northern California tested this theory with a survey completed by 572 runners and reported their findings in *Runner's World.* They observed that:

a. "Runners scoring high on stress measures also reported significantly more injuries during the past three months. Those runners had to reduce or completely skip their running more often because of injury and had more medical appointments brought about by injury. Further, the higher the stress score, the higher the scores on two illness measures: number of workdays missed and number of medical appointments brought on by illness *not* related to running injuries. These findings tended to confirm our hunch that stress adds to the risk of injury—and to other types of illness."

b. "The higher the life-change score during the past year, the greater the likelihood of running-related injuries during the past three months."

c. "There is a strong connection between injuries and chronic 'Type-A behavior'"—which the researchers define as "a pattern of time urgency, intense drive to succeed, impatience and hostility."

When faced with such stresses as marriage, divorce, a baby, lack of sleep, final exams, pressures at work, and other tensions, you must adjust your training—back off the mileage and speed work and maybe skip the big race. Take a "time out," and run just for relaxation and stress management rather than for competitive training. Otherwise, you risk not only poor performance, but serious injury or illness.

7. *Inadequate Sleep.* Fatigue tends to accumulate quickly if you don't sleep enough, leaving you feeling stale and susceptible to illness and injury. If you can't get enough sleep, for whatever reason, back off your training. Runners who overtrain frequently

develop insomnia. When the warning signs of overtraining hit you, take a break and get some rest.

Environmental Influences

1. *Bad Weather.* Beware of the obvious—slipping and falling on icy spots—as well as the not so obvious—changes in your normal footstrike and stride to adjust for poor footing in bad weather—which could cause injury. The most common winter running injuries are groin and hamstring pulls caused by slipping and sliding through the snow. The cold-weather runner is also less flexible, and thus more vulnerable to injury. Take more time to warm up properly.

Running into a strong wind or into rain or snow will lead to such injuries as shinsplints, Achilles tendinitis or an occasional stress fracture. Under these conditions the runner leans forward for long periods of time putting a strain on the anterior of the legs and on the forefoot.

2. *Surfaces and Terrain.* Ideally, your runs should take place on slightly rolling courses, without too many steep uphills or downhills. Rolling terrain gives more muscle groups a workout while not overtaxing them.

It is generally good to change surfaces frequently; however, this may cause problems for some runners. In your daily routine, don't make sudden changes in surface such as from soft to hard. A medium-hard synthetic path, a dirt trail, or even level grass fields are the best training surfaces. But if you intend to run in road races, you're going to have to run the roads for training at least a few days a week. The biggest cause of injury from running on hard pavement is not the increased shock from the surface—which is absorbed by well-cushioned shoes. Rather, it is the slant of the road. Most roads and sidewalks are banked or crowned for drainage. When you run on them, you are running along an incline; your upper foot is twisting inward with every step, and you're giving yourself a short leg. If possible, run in the middle of the road, where it is more level, or cross over the road every mile or so. Strangely, some runners find that they can run on roadbeds slanted one way but not the other.

Running on dirt trails or grass may lessen the shock to your body and strengthen muscles not used on hard surfaces. This may alleviate fatigue and injury. However, don't run on soft, uneven surfaces when injured, or you may aggravate a leg injury. The soft surface puts your legs through a greater range of motion than a hard surface. Also, avoid the temptation to run on the beach. In soft sand your heels sink in and pull your Achilles tendons. On firm, damp sand you run on a slant. Indoor running can be a blessing in the winter, but it can also cause more trouble than it is worth. Since you are running around sharp turns, often on a slanted, hard surface, you are severely stressing the inside leg and causing serious pronation on the outside leg. Limit your indoor runs to 30–45 minutes and change the direction in which you run.

Some injuries require you to run on certain surfaces. Achilles tendon problems, for example, require even, hard surfaces that don't create a pull on the damaged tendon. Knee injuries, on the other hand, are aggravated by hard surfaces. Running up or down hills may aggravate other injuries. Consult your sports-medicine expert for advice on what surfaces are best for you when fighting off an injury.

Running downhill is much more likely to cause injury than running uphill. Anyone who has ever run the Boston Marathon—known for its many downhills—realizes that running downhill in the late stages of the race causes the leg muscles, especially the quadriceps, to tighten and leaves you with sore legs for several days after. Your body absorbs much more shock on impact when running downhill, whether at training pace or racing speeds. If you "brake" going downhill, you may cause the muscles along the backs of your legs and in your back to fight against gravity, creating additional stress. Downhill running, therefore, is especially hard on those with knee or back problems. You should be relaxed and roll downhill with good form. To minimize shock, run hitting lightly on the ball of your foot and then the heel, rather than hard on the heel. And lean forward slightly as you run.

Racing downhill makes strain and stress that much more pronounced. In addition, it makes you prone to blisters and jammed toes caused by your foot sliding forward in your shoe. If you are racing or training on downhills, wear well-cushioned shoes. Avoid practicing downhill technique unless you really need it to improve your position in races. If you reach a very steep downhill during a training run, walk down it rather than risk injury.

Exercise physiologists at Oral Roberts University investigated the effects of downhill running and confirmed what most runners learn the hard way.

- Downhill running does cause muscle soreness to a much greater degree than running on the level.
- The resulting muscle soreness is accompanied by elevation of muscle enzymes in the blood. There was no elevation when the subjects ran on flat terrain. Downhill running also causes other physical changes due to the increased effort that require more time to recover from than those caused by running on level terrain.

3. *Shoes.* According to a study of over 10,000 runners by podiatrist Dr. Joe Ellis, among injured runners 71 percent blame their shoes for the injury. Ellis notes, "I do not think that shoes are the cause of most injuries. However, the runner can only blame himself, his training or his shoes. Naturally, shoes are the easiest to blame."

Running shoes designed to prevent injury often contribute to it. According to Dr. Richard Schuster, running injuries vary from year to year in response to the latest advances in running shoes.

Changes in the flexibility of the shoe and the rigidity of the heel counter, for example, may help some runners but cause problems for others. As shoes get lighter with the use of new materials, the most common breakdown is caused by weak heel counters.

To minimize injury, running shoes must offer flexibility, cushioning, and support—and they must fit your feet. Don't tie your shoes too tight, and monitor the wear of your shoes daily. Uneven wear of the soles will affect the angle of your footstrike, making your foot roll abnormally and causing injury.

Always purchase shoes from a dealer who specializes in running shoes and can help you make the right selection. Keep two pairs of training shoes going at all times to minimize injuries. This way you won't be hurt trying to get a few extra miles out of an aging pair of shoes as you break in a new one, or get blisters from having to rush new shoes into service if your trusty shoes are lost or destroyed. If you try to resole your shoes or use shoe-saving devices, be careful that you don't overcompensate and cause injury. If the midsole breaks down and loses its resiliency, don't attempt to resole the shoe; you can't replace the cushioning and support it provides.

The average competitor should use the same shoe for both racing and training. This is especially true for the heavy runner. A racing shoe gives less shock absorption and is designed for running on the ball of the foot. It also has less heel lift, and can lead to Achilles tendon injuries and shinsplints. You should wear racing shoes only for shorter races at first, and then for races beyond 10 kilometers, when you will be running much faster than your training pace. Only a few top runners can benefit from racing shoes for the marathon distance. Most runners need increased shock absorption over the 26-mile distance more than they need a little less weight. Sudden switches to spikes can also cause injury, because they have very low heels and little cushioning and they force you to run on the balls of your feet. Since most road racers would wear spikes only once or twice a year in competition, they're seldom worth the expense and injury risk.

The type of shoe you purchase may be determined by the kind of injury you are susceptible to. You may need a firm heel counter if you pronate and have a knee problem, a flexible shoe if you have shinsplints, a very well cushioned shoe if you have heel spurs, and so forth. Your sports-medicine specialist will guide you in selecting shoes to minimize your particular problem.

LISTENING TO THE WARNING SIGNS

Many running-related injuries and illnesses can be prevented, either by minimizing the causes or by paying attention to the warning signals your body sends you. The physical and mental symptoms of overstress and impending injury or illness warn you to take heed. As Dr. George Sheehan preaches, "Listen to your body, it will tell you when you are doing too much, when you are close to injury."

WARNING SIGNS CHECKLIST

Here are some of the warning signs your body may send you:

1. Mild tenderness or stiffness that doesn't go away after a day of rest or after the first few miles of your daily run.
2. A desire to quit or an unexplained poor performance in workouts and races. Also, an uncharacteristic lack of interest in training, racing, and life in general.
3. A tired feeling after a full night's sleep or a sluggish feeling that continues for several days. You may also have difficulty falling asleep, or may wake up often in the night and find it difficult to go back to sleep.
4. An increase in your morning pulse rate. Record your pulse in your diary each morning—take it when you first wake up. Note significant increases as a sign that you

haven't recovered from the previous day or days of stress. A pulse ten or more beats higher for the average runner and five or more beats higher for the highly trained runner is an indication of trouble.

5. A continued thirst despite replacement of fluids lost after your run. Check your urine. Normal urine is almost clear and odorless. A runner who is dehydrated will pass a darker urine.

6. A significant loss of body weight as measured each morning. A temporary loss of a few pounds as a result of sweating is normal. Check your weight daily and record it in your diary. A sudden loss of 2 or more pounds is not normal—fluid weight loss should be replaced by morning.

7. The feeling of a sore throat, fever, or runny nose coming on, which may indicate your susceptibility to a cold or flu. Any signs that your body is fighting infection. Also, skin blemishes and cold sores.

8. Muscle cramping caused by mineral depletion.

9. Upset stomach, diarrhea, constipation, or loss of appetite.

10. Increased irritability or feeling of tension, depression, and apathy—sure signals of the overtraining syndrome.

Respond to any of these warning signs by cutting back your mileage, minimizing or eliminating your speed work, getting more sleep, and taking off a day or two. If the symptoms persist, seek medical attention as a precaution. Don't be cheap here: You'll save on medical bills in the long run by seeking help early.

PAIN: A KEY WARNING SIGN

The most obvious warning sign is *pain*. Your body yells at you for a reason—without pain signals you would continue to train and more serious injury would result. Runners can push through *dis-*

comfort, but there's a difference between discomfort and pain. Oxygen debt and muscle fatigue are discomfort barriers. But injury and illness cause pain. Try to push through the discomfort of hard training and racing, but not through the pain signals of injury and illness. While training and racing, listen to your body, and don't try to prove your toughness by ignoring the pain you are experiencing. Also, *never* use painkillers before running. Without the sensation of pain, you could push yourself to serious injury.

Don't ignore your body's early warning signs because the pain is mild. Too many runners—especially men—feel that cutting back, resting, or taking time off makes them appear weak. Act wisely. Sometimes you can run through the stresses of competitive training and racing. But if you err, err on the side of caution. When in doubt—back off.

One helpful device is the running diary. Record your discomforts, pains, and warning signs, plus training and racing information. This will not only help you train in a consistent and injury-free pattern, but will also help you note when pain or discomfort lasts a long time. Memories on these matters are unreliable, but a detailed diary will often reveal the cause of injury and illness. Rereading your past experiences will help prevent future problems.

Perhaps the wisest way to prevent injury is occasionally to take a few days or even weeks off from serious training before major warning signs appear. By choosing to take time off, rather than being forced to by injury, you are giving your body a well-deserved rest without having to suffer physical and mental pain. You will have made an investment in your health by preventing an injury.

All injuries, however, cannot be prevented. You can only hope to minimize the possibility of injury. When it does occur, you should follow a conservative program, as detailed in Part II.

Part II

TRAINING THROUGH AND COMING BACK FROM INJURY

3
PSYCHOLOGICAL ASPECTS OF INJURY

Most runners experience some psychological difficulty when they are injured and forced to stop running. They focus on their injury and become depressed from inactivity. Few injuries last forever, though, and a runner will recover more quickly if he or she backs off and doesn't "challenge" the injury. Taking time off from running will, over the long run of your athletic career, make no difference at all. In fact, it may make you physically and mentally tougher.

For many people running has become an addiction, and when injured they experience withdrawal symptoms: insomnia, irritability, depression, tension, constipation, headaches, or muscle twinges resulting from forced inactivity. Dr. William Glasser, author of *Positive Addiction*, notes that "for those who get into running and do it on a regular basis, something builds up which is akin to an addiction. That is, if the runner doesn't run, he feels nervous, upset, anxious, tense—a tension which is relieved only by running his prescribed amount of time." Psychiatrist Dr. Kenneth E. Callen studied over 400 runners and reported in the journal *Psychosomatics* that "a striking 90 percent notice important mental or emotional benefits. . . . On the other hand, 25 percent state that they have experienced emotional problems associated with running. In almost every instance, the problem is one of depression, anger or frustration with not being able to run due to an injury."

Competitive runners also can experience negative addiction. They may lose perspective altogether, and running may become an end, not a means. The final stages of negative addiction occur when running becomes the addict's job, when family and friends are placed second, and when the addict will not stop running even when faced with serious injury. A forty-five-year-old British executive died from an overdose of aspirin. In his suicide note, he said that life was not worth living; he couldn't run because of a knee injury.

STAGES OF ADJUSTMENT FOR INJURED RUNNERS

Dr. Victor Altshul, who teaches psychiatry at the Yale University School of Medicine, wrote in *Running* magazine that those who must temporarily give up running because of an injury go through sequential emotional stages of loss similar to what one might experience with the death of a loved one. The five stages are

1. *Denial*. Often runners will not accept their injuries and will continue to run in pain until it forces them to admit they should stop.

2. *Rage*. Runners know and acknowledge that they should stop running because of an injury, but they refuse and angrily subject their bodies to more abuse. Also, they take out their frustrations on others.

3. *Depression*. After the anger subsides, runners become depressed and experience feelings of helplessness.

4. *Acceptance*. Runners accept their injuries, and they contain training within their level of tolerance. They may choose to participate in an alternative aerobic exercise to ease their depression and helplessness. They develop an intelligent plan to return gradually to their preinjury fitness level.

5. *Renewed neurotic disequilibrium*. As runners begin to re-

gain their fitness, they forget the cause of their injuries and neglect the warning signs of further injury. Too often they don't learn from their experience and once again attempt too much too soon or train for goals that are beyond their present physical and psychological capacity.

PSYCHOLOGICAL GUIDELINES FOR DEALING WITH INJURY

All runners, whether strongly or marginally addicted to running, will experience withdrawal symptoms after one to three days without exercise. According to a study at Hofstra University, approximately three-quarters of all regular runners become addicted. A Georgia State University study indicated that if habitual runners vary their schedules only slightly, negative effects result. The study revealed that when a habitual runner misses a day or two of running, he or she may feel guilty or tense.

Here are some guidelines to help you get over the blues associated with not being able to run:

1. *Accept your injury.* Analyze why it happened, and determine the causes. Treat the injury properly, seek medical attention if necessary, and develop a plan to ease back into shape.

2. *Maintain your relationships.* Don't reject your family, friends, or co-workers. Don't take out your frustrations on them or withdraw from them during your inactivity.

3. *Think positively.* Look at your injury as a scheduled rest period during your lifelong training program. Use this time to learn and enjoy alternative exercises (see Part IV). Many runners are pleasantly surprised to find after an injury that they have reached a higher level of fitness because they use the layoff time to develop upper-body strength or flexibility. They also learned to train sensibly to avoid injuries.

4. *Take a break.* Use the extra time to do things you couldn't do during your training. Take a trip with your family that isn't

dependent on a big race, or go to a baseball game with your pre–running days friends.

5. *Replace the habit, and keep active.* Maintain an active life. Activity is a powerful antidepressant. The sooner you enter another aerobic activity, the easier it will be to defeat the depression of your enforced layoff and the better shape you will be in when you are ready to resume your normal running schedule.

6. *Return to running with realistic expectations.* Be patient and conservative. You won't get it all back right away. See Chapter 5 for guidelines on coming back after a layoff.

THE PSYCHOLOGY OF HEALING

Sports psychologist Dr. Jerry Lynch stated in *The Runner:* "Once you are injured, stress can interfere with the recovery process as a result of what is known as the 'secondary illness' effect. In other words, being injured is itself stressful. . . . It takes longer to recover from the primary injury if this 'stress of being injured' is not also treated. In such a state, the body assumes a defensive posture creating, once again, physiological reactions that increase the probability of further injury. This kind of mental attitude also puts severe tension on the musculo-skeletal system, interfering with treatment efforts since muscles need to be relaxed during the healing process. The body will maintain this tense posture as long as you 'prepare for the worst,' fearful that the treatment will fail. If you perceive your prognosis as hopeful, anxiety will diminish, hastening recovery." Scientists have yet to explain how this happens but Dr. Lynch and others have had considerable success helping athletes recover from injuries by incorporating techniques of psychological stress management.

Running can be a beneficial, powerful habit. When you are not able to run because of an injury, you suffer psychological withdrawal symptoms as you decondition physically. Actively maintaining your fitness with an aerobic alternative exercise will help you cope with both the psychological and physical discomforts associated with not being able to run. Sometimes a forced layoff is good for you; it enables you to appreciate your daily exercise and makes you more conservative in your training to guard against further injury. Like many other things that are important to you, running is appreciated more when it is taken away. The lesson should be that you can cope with your depression about not being able to run and that you will return to the running trails a wiser person.

4 RUNNING THROUGH AN INJURY

The competitive runner cannot lay off every time he or she gets a minor blister, ache or pain, or sniffle. Yet by forcing yourself to continue to train, you may make thing worse. Often a day or two off will allow you to return sooner to quality training than if you had continued to aggravate your injury. Total rest beyond two or three days will not help many injuries. You may as well continue to run, or take up an alternative exercise, but within certain limits. Gentle exercise will help you maintain a base of fitness and will help you heal. The trick is to train often enough to gain these benefits while allowing the injured area to rest by doing relatively less work that does not aggravate the injury. More serious injuries or illness will require your good judgment and your doctor's advice about whether or not you should continue running, switch to an alternative exercise, or just rest. Remember, you cannot run through every injury. Listen to the pain signals your body sends you, and rely on your own experience to determine how your body reacts to injury and whether it is safe for you to run through an injury.

Joe Henderson, in his book *Run Farther, Run Faster*, listed four degrees of pain and used them as guidelines for determining whether or not you should run when injured. We have adapted his advice.

First-Degree Pain. Although it does not interfere with proper running form, you feel low-grade pain at the start of your run. The pain decreases or goes away as the run progresses, then may reappear after you stop.

Second-Degree Pain. The pain remains constant or increases slightly as your runs continue, and may remain for a few hours after. It has little effect on your running form.

Third-Degree Pain. You feel mild pain on easy runs, which gets worse as the runs progress, and severe pain on hard runs. The pain definitely interferes with proper running form. It continues after your run and usually is present throughout the day.

Fourth-Degree Pain. You cannot run without great pain and perhaps a pronounced limp.

TRAINING GUIDELINES FOR RUNNING THROUGH THE DEGREES OF PAIN

First-Degree Pain. You may be able to hold your mileage at its present level, but you should minimize speed work and long runs. Limit speed work to runs no faster than 10-kilometer race pace, and cut back the number of repetitions you would normally do. If pain starts when you do the speed work, stop and do no more until you are totally recovered. Cut back slightly on your long runs. Do not race until you can run without pain at the start of your runs. Be careful, you can get so psyched up for a race that you may not pay attention to the first-degree pain you are experiencing and may go out hard and seriously injure yourself. Don't race until you feel no pain for several days going into the event. If the pain persists after a week, cut your mileage by 25 percent and replace it with alternative aerobic exercise. It may help to alternate a day of running with a day of alternative exercises. Do not increase your mileage from its preinjury level until the pain disappears.

Second-Degree Pain. Cut your training mileage by at least 25 percent, or consider running every other day and alternating with another aerobic exercise. Eliminate the runs that cause the pain to increase, such as races, hard speed work, or hill work. You may combine your running and alternative exercise to equal your previous level of work. With your doctor's advice, you may decide that you should quit running entirely until the pain has disappeared or at least has been reduced to the first-degree level. Consider replacing running minute for minute with an aerobic alternative.

Third-Degree Pain. Start very slowly and cautiously after at least 10 minutes of brisk walking. When the pain builds up to a form-disturbing level, walk and do some easy stretching exercises for the muscle groups around the injured area. *Note:* If the muscle or tendon is inflamed, stretching it will delay the healing process. Alternate running and walking according to how you feel. The object is to keep moving and stay within the limits of safe running that your pain will set for you. At this level, you may be better off to stop running and switch to an aerobic alternative until you can run at least at the second-degree level of pain.

Fourth-Degree Pain. Stop running. Take at least one week off and do an alternative aerobic exercise. When you start again, run every other day at 50 percent of your previous mileage. If you lay off more than a week, consult the training guidelines in Chapter 5 for coming back from a layoff. If you haven't already, be sure to see a doctor.

GENERAL GUIDELINES FOR RUNNING THROUGH INJURY

• Be aware of pain and other warning signals. Pain should protect you from overdoing and developing more serious injury.

• Don't run unless you can walk briskly with little or no pain for a mile.

• Don't run if your pain makes you limp or otherwise alters your form. You may cause another injury, and it may be far worse than the one you already have.

• Run through discomfort, but not through pain. If the pain worsens as you run, stop. Your body produces its own painkilling drugs, which may allow you to run or race and forget your pain. But after the run, you may find that you have further aggravated your injury. There is a danger in pushing yourself through workouts and races which you started while in pain that disappeared after a few miles.

• Never use painkilling drugs to allow you to run. You must feel the pain so that you can adjust to it to avoid injury.

• Avoid hills, speed work, races, long runs, and slanted or soft surfaces that aggravate your injury and intensify your pain. Even if you run on a hard surface, it is better than running on uneven terrain. Some injuries will heal more quickly if you run on certain surfaces. Achilles tendon problems, for example, require hard, even surfaces that don't create a pull on the damaged tendon. Knee injuries, on the other hand, are aggravated by hard surfaces. Soft, uneven surfaces may worsen a leg injury because they put the leg through a greater range of motion than hard surfaces.

• Analyze and treat the cause of your injury. Pain is a signal. If your pain lessens when you change shoes or when you switch to the other side (and slope) of the road, you have learned its cause and can treat it.

• Make sure your shoes are right for you. They may not have adequate flexibility, cushioning, or rear foot control for your particular injury. Check with your doctor for advice. Make sure that you are not running in worn-down shoes—in fact, they may have contributed to the injury in the first place.

• Consult Chapter 16 for advice about treating your injury.

• Check Chapter 14 for information about aids that can be used to help keep you on the running paths. Heel lifts can help you run through minor problems with shinsplints, Achilles tendinitis, and other lower-leg problems. Pads taped to appropriate places on your feet can help you run through pains in the heel and ball of the foot. Products such as 2d Skin can be used to cover blisters and allow you to keep running. Commercial orthotics and taping techniques can help you continue running despite such problems as knee pain, heel spurs, and plantar fasciitis.

• If you wear orthotics, the first thing you should do if you develop an injury is check with your doctor to see if an adjustment in the device will help you run through and eliminate the injury.

• Warm up and cool down thoroughly with each run.

• Do specific exercises to strengthen or improve flexibility. They will help heal your injury and prevent further occurrence. See Chapter 17 for exercises that can help rehabilitate some specific injuries. Do not overstretch or stretch injured parts until they have recovered.

• Adjust your training if need be. Run twice a day for less time or distance to get in mileage with less continuous pounding and aggravation to the injury. For example, two runs a day of 5 miles each may allow you to run pain-free even though you would develop pain after 7 miles during a 10-mile run. Plan ahead to run for three or four days and then take a day off to allow your body to rebuild and keep ahead of breakdown. Run up to the edge of your capacity, and then, before you feel pain, walk briskly. Continue to alternate running and walking for 4 to 5 miles.

• Be patient, and persevere.

The key to running through your injury is to develop a feel for your limits. If during a training run you aggravate an injury or develop one that causes you to change your form or is painful, stop and ask for a ride home or take a cab. Don't force yourself to run a few more miles so that you can keep on schedule. During a race or speed workout, if you feel an injury or tightness coming on, stop. Don't be foolish and push yourself to finish; you'll be a hero today and a fool in pain tomorrow.

Distance runners sometimes develop high tolerances for pain. This probably means that they are good at putting up with the discomfort of low-level pain, but are aware of it and adjust or train accordingly. All runners must develop a sense of their limits. This may mean, for example, running up to 5 miles before the knee acts up and later increasing to 7 miles as the knee strengthens. Since you are the one experiencing the pain, only you can determine the limits of training you can handle. You must balance the need to continue in order to build or maintain fitness with the need to prevent destruction of your health—and thus your training. Better to play the limits wisely than to challenge those limits and risk long-term setback.

5 COMING BACK FROM A LAYOFF

When a runner is unable to run through an injury and is forced to stop training, he or she is faced with three considerations: How much conditioning did I lose during the layoff? How long will it take me to return to my previous level of fitness? How can I train for the comeback both to regain lost fitness and to minimize the chances of reinjury?

DETRAINING

How quickly will performance be affected after you stop training? According to physiologist David Costill in *The Runner*, "In general, there is no loss in performance for five to seven days. As a matter of fact, running performance may even be improved after two to four days of inactivity. Such 'rest' periods allow the muscles and nervous system to recover and rebuild from the stress of heavy training, thereby providing the runner with improved reserves and greater tolerance for endurance exercises." The point to learn here is clear: Don't panic if you need to miss a *few* days of training to baby an injury or illness; you will not lose the conditioning you have built up.

But when you are unable to train for more than a few days, you lose your conditioning fast. Various studies show that fitness is lost two to three times as fast as it is gained. Studies show that a healthy marathon runner who loses ten days of training will lose 10 percent of his or her endurance. According to Costill, not training at all for eight or ten weeks will result in the loss of 80 to

100 percent of the conditioning gains. Whether injured or ill, you will need two or three days of rehabilitation training for every day lost. Even if you were in racing shape when you stopped running, it generally takes two weeks of easy aerobic endurance training plus a week of sharpening training, including speed work, for every week lost before you can return to a preinjury level of fitness. If you lay off a month, you may need nine to twelve weeks to return to your level of conditioning. If you are concerned about keeping the racing edge, you can significantly shorten the time required to return to preinjury condition if you replace your running time minute for minute with an aerobic equivalent.

A complete layoff of several weeks will result in atrophy or loss of muscle size, loss of strength, loss of endurance, loss of flexibility and coordination, and loss of mental confidence. When you lay off, you will feel a sense of loss, and you may become cranky, but a layoff can be a blessing in disguise. You will appreciate the joys of being able to run, and it will stimulate you to set new goals and go out to attain them. In fact, during your layoff you should establish two goals for yourself: a return to your previous fitness level, and an improvement in your time.

COMING BACK

The amount of time it takes to come back depends on how long you've been off, what alternative workouts you have done, and what put you out in the first place. Each injury or illness has its own special road to recovery. A minor cold, for example, will allow you to return to light running at a slow pace within a day or so. A more serious flu or injury will obviously take longer. When you are feeling better, plan your recovery program. The loss of a week or two may require only a week or two of gradually progressive training, starting at one-third to one-half the preinjury distance. Longer layoffs for more serious injuries require a more conservative comeback. Plan to return after long layoffs by alternating running and walking in a program similar to a beginner's except that you can progress more quickly since you can return in less time than you needed to build up when you started. Also take days off between running days. Start slowly. You'll feel side stitches, wobbly knees, muscle soreness, weakness. Be careful. Veteran runners often find that their heart and lungs can return much faster than their musculoskeletal system, and that they are more vulnerable to muscle strain and injury than they expected. Dr. Steve Subotnik noted in *The Running Foot Doctor,* "I have . . . found that bone has a tendency to lose its strength after a lay-off of two to three weeks, making it more susceptible to stress fractures. I caution everyone who has had an injury which has laid them up for much over two weeks to take it really easy when returning to running. The body adapts to stress rapidly and becomes desensitized to stresses rapidly." This would hold true both for the runner who completely stops training and for the person who uses alternative, non-weight-bearing exercises while laying off from running. Dr. Subotnik also noted, "Runners have to realize that it takes a long time to totally rehabilitate themselves. When runners finally acknowledge this, maybe they'll begin laying off a little sooner instead of continuing to run with pain. . . . It takes as long to get healthy after an injury as it took to get the injury." That is, if you felt the pain in your ankle two months ago, kept running, and got hurt, you'll spend two months getting well. Once again: Listen to the warning signs your body gives you.

TRAINING GUIDELINES FOR COMING BACK FROM ILLNESS AND INJURY

Coming Back from Illness

Each type of illness requires a different treatment and different training method for recovery. A slight cold may be helped by short runs at a slow pace. Flu, accompanied by fever, dizziness, severe weakening, and a loss of desire to run, demands complete rest. Never begin a program of recovery training until the illness is well under control.

Tom Osler detailed a plan for recovery from illness in his booklet, *The Conditioning of Distance Runners*. He wrote: "Let us suppose that the athlete has suffered a minor virus infection, and has rested for about five days. He may still have a few sniffles, but no coughing or fever. After deciding that his body definitely has the problem under control (he is no longer taking medication), he should try the following recovery plan, designed to return him to reasonable fitness in seven days: The runner should divide the length of his medium runs by seven. He will run this distance very slowly the first day. Symptoms of side stitch, muscle soreness, and weakness are likely to be felt. The second day the runner should try to add one seventh of his medium run to the first day's mileage, again running easy. He should observe that he feels much better than he did the day before. If he does not, he should return to complete rest, for he is not prepared for running. Each day he adds one seventh of the medium run to his previous day's mileage, running it at an easy relaxed pace. He must continually observe the sensation that although he is running farther, it is easier. After seven days he will probably feel ready to resume normal training.

"In the event that the athlete has suffered a more serious illness, he should consider a more gradual return to fitness in perhaps two or three weeks or longer. It may be necessary in extreme cases to begin with walking. In any case, the distance should slowly be increased according to a plan similar to that described above. Daily improvement must be observed, or a return to rest is demanded. In no case should the athlete attempt fast running until complete recovery is established."

Coming Back from Injury
All runners at all levels of fitness must be very conservative when coming back from a layoff. As previously noted, losing a

week or two may require only a week or two of gradually progressive training starting at one-third to one-half the preinjury distance per day. For example, if you were averaging 5 miles a day and laid off entirely for a full week because of shinsplints, your recovery program might look like this: Day 1: Run 2 miles; Day 2: Run 3 miles; Day 3: Run 4 miles; Day 4: Off; Day 5: Run 4 miles; Day 6: Run 4 miles; Day 7: Run 5 miles.

After a layoff of two weeks or more, you should start with a goal of 3–5 miles, alternating running and walking. The longer the time you laid off and the more severe the injury, the less time you should spend running nonstop before taking a walk break. If you had been averaging 50 miles a week and had laid off for six weeks because of a stress fracture, you might use the following recovery program. Remember to walk briskly at least 10 minutes before each run. Day 1: Run for 3 minutes followed by brisk walking for 3 minutes until 3 miles are covered; Day 2: Repeat; Day 3: Off; Day 4: Run for 5 minutes followed by brisk walking for 3 minutes; Day 5: Repeat; Day 6: Off; Day 7: Run for 1 mile followed by 2 minutes of brisk walking and repeat two times; Day 8: Run for 1½ miles followed by 2 minutes of brisk walking and repeat once; Day 9: Off; Day 10: Run for 3 miles; Day 11: Repeat; Day 12: Run for 4 miles; Day 13: Off; Day 14: Run for 5 miles. From this point on you would return to running an average of 5 miles a day for six days of running, taking one day off each week.

SPECIFIC GUIDELINES FOR COMING BACK FROM INJURY

Adapt these four principal guidelines to your particular situation:

1. Slowly increase the running period and decrease the walking period until you can run nonstop comfortably for a 3- to 5-mile distance.
2. Slowly build back up to your normal training base; never increase your distance by more than 10 percent a week.

3. Don't attempt hills, long runs, or speed work until you have run at least two weeks at your previous distance level.
4. Jogging very slowly may aggravate your injury or cause another from altered form. Thus, it may be better to run a fairly normal pace and take walk breaks to prevent continuous pounding.

Other useful guidelines include the following:

- Reach the base your body can tolerate, and stay there until you feel strong. That might be 40 miles a week instead of the 60 miles that caused the breakdown. Learn your limits, and gradually increase your base. Consider replacing some of the extra mileage, which may cause injury, with an aerobic alternative.
- If you lost a day or two to minor injury or a cold, don't try to make them up. Pick up where you can on your normal schedule as soon as it is safe.
- Don't run if your form is altered because you are favoring an injury while on the comeback trail. You could cause a new injury, which might even be worse than your original problem.
- Be patient. Periodic "testing" of the injury by trying to run farther or faster than your conservative recovery schedule calls for may result in reinjury and the loss of even more training time.
- Set goals well below your threshold of further injury. Avoid frustration. Give yourself the satisfaction of making slow and steady progress.
- Approach your racing goals differently. Run the first few races after your layoff just to experience racing again. Next, aim to approach your prelayoff times, and then to match and exceed them. But don't be in a hurry.
- Reanalyze again and again the *cause* of your injury or illness. Learn from your mistakes and don't repeat them.

USING ALTERNATIVE TRAINING

If you use alternative aerobic exercises while forced off the running trails by injury, you can come back to running much faster. In this case your concern is not so much cardiovascular detraining, but rather the ability of your musculoskeletal system—particularly the injured area—to handle the pounding of running after a layoff. This problem would be minimized if you were able to walk, race walk, or cross-country ski, because these are weight-bearing activities. However, many serious injuries require non-weight-bearing exercise such a swimming or biking. Here are some guidelines to follow for returning to full-time running:

- Throughout your recovery process maintain the aerobic equivalent of the level you were at before the injury. Thus, if you were running 30–60 minutes a day, you should combine your aerobic alternative with running (if you *can* run) to average 30–60 minutes of aerobic work per day.

- Return to running following a program similar to that for a runner coming back from a complete layoff caused by injury. You may choose to start with 15–20 minutes of running nonstop at an easy pace rather than the run-walk system. Add your aerobic workout (swimming, for example) before or after your run to complete a 30–60 minute workout. On the off days, swim for 30–60 minutes. Listen to your body, and gradually replace your aerobic alternative with running as you return to your preinjury level.

- During the entire recovery phase, and for at least two weeks after you start running your normal mileage, replace speed work—if you need it to prepare for key races—with anaerobic work in the pool or on the bike. Also, do your long runs—if you need them to prepare for a marathon—with a combination of running and an aerobic alternative. For example, you might build up to running for an hour and then swim or bicycle for another hour to complete the aerobic equivalent of a 2-hour run, protecting your body from excessive pounding.

SUCCESS STORIES

If you feel discouraged because you can't run, perhaps you will feel better knowing that even the greatest runners get injured, stop running, and come back to the top.

Angella Hearn, a member of the Atalanta Women's Running Team, is a good example of a runner who was determined to come back after an injury and succeeded. She was highly motivated to do so; both she and her identical-twin sister, Chris, were scheduled to return home to England to run the 1982 London Marathon—the first marathon they planned to run together and their first race in England. After running the October 1981 New York Marathon in 2:53, Angella began feeling a twinge on the inner side of one lower shin. Four months later it became much worse, and she was advised to stop running for several weeks. It was three months before the London Marathon, and she was training 80 miles per week. She was determined to continue training for London and, as her coach, Bob Glover directed her to the swimming pool, where she had developed a rigorous program to fit her needs.

She swam for one hour each morning before work and for one-half hour each evening after work for four full weeks. In her six-day-a-week program she didn't run a step, yet she included speed work to sharpen her fitness work.

After a month without running, Angella began a two-week program that included the hour swim each morning but replaced her evening swims with some easy runs. She began with a run around the block, just to get the feel of running again. The goal was to return to running slowly to avoid aggravating the injury. She really had to discipline herself, because her heart and lungs were strong enough to allow her to run much farther and faster than her injury could tolerate. Within two weeks after she started running again, she gradually moved from running 2 miles a day to running 5 miles a day. She cut her swimming training back to twice a week just for the speed work because she still couldn't do that safely by running. From there she moved up to running 8-mile runs alternated with days consisting of two 5-mile runs.

Six weeks before the marathon she was again running 70 miles a week, but being careful not to stress the injury.

Long runs were then extended weekly to 13, 16, and 18 miles and then to a single 20-miler. No speed work was done outside the pool until one month before the marathon, when Angella ran a few half-mile sessions at marathon pace to get a feel for racing again. She ran one 10-kilometer race two weeks before London to prove to herself that the leg would hold up to the stress.

During this entire period, Angella did weight training three times a week to keep her upper body, quadriceps, and abdominals fit for racing. She also did special exercises to strengthen the muscles in the shin area, where she was injured. In addition, she had ultrasound treatments every other day, which helped speed up recovery time, and she had her orthotics adjusted. Finally, she altered her footstrike temporarily from ball-heel to heel-ball to minimize the strain on the lower leg.

Before her injury Angella had been aiming for a 2:45 marathon. Most runners would have given up hope of being able even to finish a marathon after losing two full months of normal training. Angella modified her goals and was triumphant before her family and friends by completing the May 1982 London Marathon in a personal record of 2:50:05. Her sister, inspired by Angella's dedication, ran a 2:56:55 in her marathon debut.

In the spring of 1980 Alberto Salazar was so badly hurt that he had to stop running and swam for training for a few weeks. Then, after only a few weeks back on his feet, he qualified for the U.S. Olympic team for 10 kilometers. He was injured again in the summer, but returned to win his first ever marathon in New York in 1981. He came back the following year to set a world record of 2:08:13.

Norway's Grete Waitz could not run a step for three weeks in July 1982 because of a stress fracture. She kept in shape by riding an indoor bike at high resistance for a half-hour each day. When she resumed running, she started back slowly, with only 15 minutes of easy running each day. By the fifth day she was running for 35 minutes, and by the eleventh day she had resumed her normal training. About a week later her quads became very tight; her body told her she was coming back too fast, so she backed off again. Gradually, she returned to fitness and won the New York Marathon in October, three months after resuming running. The following spring she tied the world marathon record with a big win in the London Marathon in 2:25:29, and that summer she convincingly won the first women's marathon in the World Championship in Helsinki.

In late December 1981 Joan Benoit was operated on for injury to both Achilles tendons. Two days later, wearing walking casts on each leg, she started riding an indoor bike for 30–45 minutes daily against good resistance. She also added very demanding speed work on the bike to keep her competitive edge. She started running again the first of March. Ten weeks later she set an American record for 25 kilometers. Then in September 1982, less than seven months after resuming running, she set an American women's marathon record of 2:26:11 at the Nike Marathon in Eugene, Oregon.

Benoit wrote in the 1982 New York Marathon program: "high mileage should never be a goal in itself. When I first started competing in the marathon, I found myself running a lot of unnecessary mileage for no reason other than to be able to write bigger and bigger numbers in my diary. I didn't take the time to think things through until I was forced to take 10 weeks off this past winter.

"It was at this point that I decided to cut back on my running and include alternative exercises in my training. Bicycling, swimming and weight training have now replaced the excessive mileage that served no constructive purpose. These other activities have allowed me to enjoy running more than ever, since I am refreshed and eager when I do step out on the roads."

The following spring she demolished the world record by over 2 minutes with a 2:22:42 Boston Marathon victory.

Benoit made an even more remarkable comeback from an injury in 1984. In March she developed a knee problem which caused her to miss a significant amount of training leading up to the first ever Women's Olympic Marathon Trials in May. She tried alternating days of running with days of rest and even cortisone shots. In mid-April she tried one last step before submitting to surgery—she took the powerful anti-inflammatory drug, butazolidin, and rested for five days. Seventeen days before the Trials she submitted to arthroscopic surgery. Dr. Stan James, an orthopedic surgeon, discovered that she had a plica band in her right knee that was too tight, and snipped it. Almost immediately after surgery she started on a program of rehabilitation. First she pedaled a bike with her arms while lying on her back, then she walked on a treadmill. Five days later she ran 55 minutes in the morning and 60 in the afternoon. Within five days she couldn't run at all because of an extremely tight left hamstring—an injury caused by compensating for the injured right knee. She was given special treatment with an acuscope, which sends electronic charges to the injured areas and re-establishes electrical activity. A week later, only 17 days after knee surgery, Benoit won the Olympic Trials Marathon in Olympia, Washington, in 2:31:04. Three months later she won the Olympic gold medal in the marathon (the first Olympic marathon ever for women) in Los Angeles in 2:24:46.

Part III
THE AFTERMARATHON

6 PREVENTING INJURY AFTER RUNNING THE MARATHON

Thousands of runners each year put in hundreds of hours of physical and mental preparation to run the marathon. Very little time or planning, however, is devoted to what happens after the marathon. The scene at the finish line of a major marathon resembles a disaster area. The marathon tears down the body, which has been built up for months in anticipation of a strong effort. Injury and illness are frequent not only during and immediately after the marathon, but also in the days and weeks following. The body is weak, and the mind is undisciplined because the immediate goal has been achieved. A postmarathon runner is very vulnerable. How well you recover from a marathon effort and prevent injury from developing depends on how effectively you deal with the three key phases of marathon recovery:

1. Your prerace preparation
2. *Race day* strategy and execution, and environmental influences
3. *Postrace* recovery procedures and training for several weeks following the marathon

Both Bob Glover and Dr. Weisenfeld see many runners come down with injuries resulting from carelessness in the "after-marathon" period. Because we feel that most runners seriously neglect the not-so-glamorous days following the excitement of a marathon, we want to call attention to that period here by devoting a full chapter to it.

PRERACE PREPARATION

Training. The better trained you are for the marathon, the better your chances of a healthy, quick recovery. The first-time marathon runner who builds to a minimum of 40–50 miles per week will take longer to recover fully and will be more vulnerable to injury than the veteran marathoner who logs 60–70 miles per week. Another factor is the frequency of long runs in the three to four months before a marathon. At least two runs a month of 18–20 miles will train the body to race better—and recover from—the marathon event. Runners who intend to race faster than their daily training pace also need to put in some speed work and run shorter races at marathon pace or faster to prepare their bodies for the stresses of racing at a strong pace over distance. A proper tapering program will not only help you run a faster race, but also help you recover faster and minimize injury. A rested, fresh body is less prone to injury when subjected to the rigors of a marathon race.

Remember this key point: Most injuries during the build-up stage are a result of overtraining; many injuries during the marathon and the postmarathon period are caused by undertraining. If you feel that you may not be properly trained for a good marathon effort, then wait for next year's event, when you will be more likely to run faster and emerge from the marathon uninjured.*

Prerace Injury. Stubbornly starting a marathon with an injury could make the injury far worse or create another even more serious than the first one. The officials of New York Marathon, aware

---

* *The Competitive Runner's Handbook* details a complete twenty-six week build-up schedule for first-time marathoners and eighteen-week build-up schedules for veterans.

that runners would do anything to compete in their event, started a policy in 1982 that allows runners to cancel because of injury or undertraining and be guaranteed entry into the race the following year. In 1984 over 2,500 of 18,000 original accepted applicants took advantage of this offer. Over one-half of those surveyed said that if it had not been for this policy they would have tried to compete, even though they were injured, rather than pass up the opportunity to participate in this highly publicized event. If you take a chance and start a marathon with an injury, the odds are high than you'll be a double loser. You'll run poorly, if not be forced to drop out; and you'll be laid up with the injury for several weeks or more, thus losing out on future racing goals.

Racing Weight. The more you weigh, the more force you hit the ground with at each footstrike. The more you weigh above your ideal racing weight, the greater your chances of becoming injured during or after the marathon.

Flexibility and Muscle Balance. Poor flexibility and muscle imbalance will affect your recovery rate. The marathon severely taxes relatively weak muscles, such as the quadriceps, and tightens the muscles primarily used in running, the antigravity muscles in the back and legs. If you experience tightness in your hamstrings before the marathon begins, you will be prone to injury after the event.

Age and Experience. Marathon runners peak out physically somewhere between the ages of twenty-five and thirty-five. You might still be able to improve your times after that, but most people start slowing down after age thirty-five. Another major consideration for older marathoners is recovery. The older you are the longer your body takes to recover adequately and thus the greater your danger in trying to come back to hard training and racing after a marathon effort.

For the most part, the more marathons you have run the easier it is to recover and the less prone you are to injury. This is not only because you are in better shape, but because you have learned valuable lessons about how to listen to your body's warning signs during the critical rebuilding periods after your previous marathons.

Prerace-day Food. The marathon runner utilizes glycogen—carbohydrates stored in the muscles and liver—for his or her primary source of fuel. The average, well-trained runner can store enough glycogen to last approximately 20 miles, at which point he or she begins to fatigue suddenly, "hitting the wall," and has to depend on slower-burning fat for fuel. The earlier a runner "hits the wall," the more fatigued and the more vulnerable to illness and injury he or she will be after the race. A marathoner can increase glycogen storage and minimize the tearing-down effect of glycogen depletion by carbohydrate loading: For the three days before the marathon include a high percentage of carbohydrates in your diet. Be sure to eat some protein, but don't overeat. And get plenty of rest. This procedure, explained in detail in *The Competitive Runner's Handbook*, increases the amount of glycogen stored in your body prior to a marathon.

Prerace-day Fluid Intake. For two weeks before the race drink plenty of water, especially the last few days as you load with carbohydrates. Water is needed in correct balance to keep the body healthy; an even greater quantity of water is needed when you are carbohydrate loading because extra fluid is required to store the added glycogen properly.

RACE DAY PREPARATION

Correct Pacing. If you start too fast, you'll suffer much more at the end of the marathon than if you run an evenly paced race. Start no more than 10–15 seconds per mile faster than the pace you realistically expect to average for the race. A properly paced race will significantly minimize damage to your body and speed up the recovery process.

Proper Form. Errors in running form cause many injuries. The impact of these form faults is greatly magnified when repeated over and over during 3–5 hours of hard running. Even someone with good running form can lose control of it in the late stages of a race when fatigue, glycogen depletion, and—if the race isn't going well—depression can combine to produce running form errors that could make the runner more vulnerable to injuries following the marathon by overtaxing key parts of the musculoskeletal system. Attempt to concentrate on proper form even when you are fatigued so you can improve your race time, increase recovery time, and minimize injury. If—because of extreme fatigue—your form in the late stages of the marathon and your race pace are very poor, seriously consider dropping out to protect yourself from losing a lot of training time as a result of injury.

Injury. As with extreme fatigue, if you are losing good form because of injury you are liable to cause further injury. Drop out! Swallow your pride and use common sense. Consider this: One runner in the New York Marathon continued running through pain until she was forced to stop when her leg broke less than a half-mile from the finish line. Respect pain, don't be afraid to drop out to prevent serious injury and/or an extended loss of training time. Be especially careful of continuing to run while favoring painful blisters.

Shoes. Well-cushioned training shoes protect you better from pounding than racing shoes—especially on downhills. They also have higher heels, which minimize strain on the Achilles tendons, shins, and calves. If you insist on wearing racing shoes in an attempt to race a fast marathon, be aware that it may take you longer to recover. The average marathoner is better off opting for protection from injury rather than lightness of the shoe.

Heat. The lingering effects of dehydration during a hot marathon will make you vulnerable to injury. You can minimize this danger by starting slower and adjusting your race goal. If you start fast and unrealistically challenge the heat, you'll pay for it for several weeks.

Wind. Strong head winds wear you down and slow not only your time, but your recovery as well. They also make you lean forward, taxing the lower legs even more. Bob Glover fought strong head winds for over 20 miles in the 1983 Long Island Marathon—his first in five years—and his recovery time was slowed by a full two weeks. Beware once again of coming back too strong when coming off a marathon that presented you with special weather hazards on top of the challenge of racing 26.2 miles.

Hills. Hilly courses, particularly those with several steep downhills, cause extra damage to your muscles. You have to be especially careful when recovering from races such as the Boston Marathon, noted for its downhills. Cold, wet weather combined with downhills causes the muscles to become even more stiff and prone to injury.

Fluids. It is very important—in order to minimize the dangers of dehydration and improve recovery time—to be adequately hydrated before and during the marathon. The American College of Sports Medicine recommends that runners drink 13–17 ounces of fluids 10–15 minutes before racing (or for that matter before long runs). Normally your kidneys shut down as you start running, so last-minute fluid intake that doesn't reach the kidneys will remain in your body. Thus, you are actually "fluid loading." This extra fluid will be immediately available for sweat, which helps cool the body on a hot day. It will also help prevent or delay dehydration and overheating.

Look for water stations at the starting area. Water is your safest bet before the race.

The body loses fluids more rapidly than they can be absorbed through the stomach. On hot days, you should drink more than you think is necessary. Don't rely on your thirst: You could be down 1–2 quarts of sweat before your mouth even feels thirsty.

Drink as much as you can without upsetting your stomach—a further reason for drinking mainly water. According to Dr. David Costill, exercise physiologist and author of *A Scientific Approach to Distance Running*, "During the marathon, you can't even come close to replacing the fluids you lose. Drinking at aid stations may replace only one tenth of the fluids you lose. But this 10 percent is important."

Start drinking about 10–15 minutes before the beginning of the race, and then drink about every 15 minutes during the race on hot days (somewhat less often on cool days). Fluid stations should be located about every 2 miles. Your body can absorb about 6 ounces of fluid every 15–20 minutes. Therefore, you should take a full cup of liquid every 2 to 3 miles. It takes up to 20 minutes for the fluid to be absorbed and take effect, so don't wait until you feel hot and thirsty to begin drinking. By then it will be too late. Fluids consumed during the last 2 or 3 miles may not help you in your race, but they will aid in your recovery.

POSTRACE RECOVERY

Immediately after finishing the marathon you must fight the urge to lie down and give up the hope that your pain and fatigue will go away. Force yourself to begin the very important but largely neglected postrace recovery process. If you fail to take care of your aching body properly after the marathon, your legs will soon become very tight and you will be extremely prone to injury over the next few days and weeks of running.

This is the postrace recovery procedure that is most effective in helping runners to recover safely and quickly:

The First Hours. Keep moving when you finish the race. Don't lie or sit down for long periods of time. If you do sit down, try to keep your feet elevated. After leaving the chute, drink plenty of fluids, put on warm-ups, walk. Then get off your feet for a few minutes and drink some more fluids. Have any blisters treated immediately by medical personnel at the finish area. Apply ice to any painful areas in the major leg muscle groups, and repeat the process along with taking aspirin for the next few days to combat inflammation. It is the swelling around the traumatized muscles that causes soreness and tightness. Do some very light stretching, but don't overstretch fatigued muscles.

We recommend that you avoid heat treatment of the painful areas for 48 hours. However, some people find that a hot bath or whirlpool bath will relax them. If you do take a hot bath, treat the injured area with ice first. After the bath, take a short nap or at least lie down and rest. After you have gained some strength, go for a 10–15 minute walk and eat some food.

Later in the day, go for another walk (15–30 minutes), swim, ride a bike, or go dancing. The purpose of this activity is to pump blood into the legs in order to help flush away the waste products that have accumulated. Force yourself to do the unnatural—exercise when your body doesn't want to. Apply more ice and stretch some more before going to bed.

Fluids. Start replacing fluids as soon as you cross the finish line. Sip fluids if you cannot gulp them. When your stomach settles, pour them in. In hot weather consume cold drinks to bring down your body temperature as well as replace the fluid loss. In cold weather also drink some cold water to replace lost fluids, but then add something warm to prevent chill.

You should drink plenty of fluids throughout the day in proportion to the amount of weight you lost. An average runner might lose as much as 8 pounds of water weight running a marathon. Keep drinking until you have clear urine; dark urine is a symptom of dehydration. Force yourself to drink extra fluids. Watch your body weight for the next 24 hours. Generally this is enough time to get your fluids—and your weight—back to normal.

Beware of chronic dehydration, which can be caused by going

several days without properly replenishing lost fluids. This is a dangerous condition that is frequently overlooked. It lowers a runner's tolerance to fatigue, reduces the ability to sweat, elevates the rectal temperature, and increases stress on the circulatory system. According to Dr. David Costill, "Probably the best way to guard against chronic dehydration is to check your weight every morning before breakfast. If you note a two or three pound decrease in body weight from morning to morning, efforts should be made to increase your fluid intake. You need not worry about drinking too much fluid, because your kidneys will unload the excess water in a matter of hours." According to Dr. Edward Colt, "There is a lot of evidence that runners are suffering from chronic dehydration which becomes even more severe during long runs or marathons. The evidence for this is the sixfold increase in kidney stones among marathon runners which Paul Milvy, John Thorton and I reported in the *Journal of Sports Medicine and Physical Fitness.* Kidney stones occur much more frequently in people who are dehydrated. Susceptibility to urine infections also results."

Food. Runners who are obsessed with proper diet before a race often ignore it afterward. But what you eat and drink for several days after a marathon will affect your recovery. A balanced diet, with an emphasis on carbohydrates, will replenish all your energy stores of fat and glycogen and allow you to return sooner to a normal training and racing routine.

A marathon will especially deplete your glycogen stores. To recover, and to replace lost glycogen, you should eat plenty of carbohydrates. In effect, this is a carbohydrate reloading to get glycogen back into your muscles and liver. Dr. Costill says, "Probably the first meal after the marathon should be like the last big meal before. You want to recover as much of that used-up glycogen as possible. It often takes three to five days to recover the glycogen. That's part of the problem of recovering from a marathon. A lot of people don't go after the carbohydrates hard enough, and that is part of the cause for the fatigue and difficulties in getting back into running form again."

The Days Following the Marathon

Joe Henderson commented in his book *Run Farther, Run Faster*, "Recovery seems to go backward at first. You feel worse the morning after the race than you did right after, and worse yet the second day. It takes that long for the 'drunk' to wear off, and the soreness and fatigue to settle in completely. You typically hit bottom about forty-eight hours after racing. You aren't tempted to do much running in this state, and you aren't thinking much about racing again. After another twenty-four to forty-eight hours pass, the worst of the hurts disappear. You think you're ready to start training for another race, but that's where you're wrong—perhaps dangerously wrong. Recovery isn't finished when your legs loosen up; it has only begun.

"Racing tears you down in more ways than one. I see at least three stages of recovery. They are: (1) muscular, (2) chemical, and (3) psychological. Recovery from muscle soreness and fatigue comes quickest. Even marathoners get over it within a few days. But it takes longer to restore body chemistry to its normal balance, and still longer to forget how bad this race felt so you can start looking forward to the next one."

Here are general guidelines and a sample program to follow for the first week following a marathon.

• The morning after the marathon take another bath to relax, but remember to treat injured areas with ice first. Do more gentle stretching, and take a walk or easy run. You may be better off forgetting about running for a few days. Stick to non-weight-bearing exercise, such as swimming or biking. The object is to recover by forcing blood into the legs to remove waste products, so why abuse the body by compelling it to run on blistered feet and tired legs?

• Treat injured areas with ice for the first 48 hours. You may later use heat treatments such as whirlpool baths or ultrasound and massage to promote circulation. Do gentle stretching exercises in the first 48 hours, and be cautious—remember, your muscles will be tight.

SAMPLE PROGRAM FOR ONE WEEK FOLLOWING A MARATHON

Monday	Walk for 30 minutes in the morning; swim or bike for 30 minutes in the evening.
Tuesday	Walk for 30 minutes in the morning; swim or bike for 30 minutes in the evening.
Wednesday	Walk for 15 minutes and then run for 15–30 minutes in the morning; swim or bike for 30 minutes in the evening.
Thursday	*Run 4–6 miles easy**
Friday	Run 4–6 miles easy
Saturday	Run 4–8 miles with a few brisk pickups of 100 yards at 10-kilometer pace.
Sunday	Run your average medium-distance day—approximately 6–10 miles.

* If you find it difficult to run with good form because of injury or tight muscles, continue to use aerobic alternatives until you can comfortably run again.

• Get plenty of sleep for several days after your big race. Go to bed early, and take naps if possible. It is extremely important to get much more than the normal amount of sleep.

• Beware of a false high you may experience a few days after a strong marathon effort. Hold back. Even though you feel as if you are very strong, you are not. Also be careful following a disappointing race not to punish yourself by running hard in an effort to improve immediately for your next race.

REBUILDING—THE NEXT FEW WEEKS

Recovery is your priority for two weeks or more after the marathon. By the third week you may be able to run your normal mileage. Don't rush it. Recovery can take four to eight weeks, and it deserves as much planning as your premarathon schedule. Besides recovering from muscle soreness, you need time to restore your body chemistry to its normal balance and time for you again to desire to train properly for your next race. First-time marathoners and those who run behind the middle of the pack shouldn't race any distance for five to eight weeks after the marathon; advanced marathoners shouldn't race for four to six weeks.

Part IV
ALTERNATIVE TRAINING

7

HOW TO CHOOSE AND USE ALTERNATIVE AEROBIC TRAINING

Alternative aerobic training is one of the least used and most valuable aspects of a runner's training program. We consider it an essential aid to runners who can't run because of injury, are coming back from injury, or wish to prevent injury.

OPTIONS FOR THE INJURED RUNNER WHO CAN'T RUN

You have four options when you are injured and can't run.

Take Time Off. Taking time off is the simplest option—merely rest. This is the best choice for a few days while a minor injury mends or an illness such as the flu runs its course. But if you are like most runners, you will want to do some exercise to keep fit and to chase away the feeling of depression associated with not running. Alternative aerobic exercise is the answer.

Maintain Absolute Minimal Fitness. If you know it will be more than a few days before you'll be able to run again—especially if you have to lay off for two weeks or more—you may, if your doctor agrees, choose to do some type of alternative aerobic exercise three to five times a week for 30 consecutive minutes each time. This will maintain minimal cardiovascular and musculoskeletal fitness and prepare you to come back sooner. You may also find the easier schedule a mental relief. You may lose considerable fitness from the competitive level, though, so don't press too hard during your return.

Replace Running with an Alternative Exercise. To maintain near-normal fitness when forced off the running trails, you should try to replace your running minute for minute with alternative aerobic exercise. Check with your doctor to make sure you can safely do the new activity. Build gradually to the same amount of *time* you had spent running: for example, one hour a day. If possible, this training should be done at the same vigorous level of exertion as running to achieve aerobic benefit. This option will allow you to replace the running habit psychologically, and, although you'll lose some fitness, you will also be able to return to running in good shape.

Impersonate a Competitive Runner. If you really *have* to be ready for a big race, then only lack of imagination and discipline need stop you. This is the top level, the serious runner who has to lay off running for a while but can still exercise vigorously. Build up slowly, follow the hard-easy system, and include training specific to your goals. The same principles that apply to competitive running apply here. If you are in a build-up stage, long bike rides or swims will build strength and endurance. Build up to the time you would spend on your long runs, or longer. All types of speed workouts can be done on a bike, in the pool, and so on if you need to sharpen close to a race. Later, as you begin to run again, you may be able to do aerobic running without risking injury but choose to continue doing your speed work with an alternative exercise, or complete your long run with a combination of running for a medium-length distance followed immediately by some additional training in an alternative activity. Examples of speed workouts that can be used with alternative training are included in Chapters 8 and 9, on biking and swimming respectively.

COMING BACK FROM INJURY

Alternative aerobic exercises—especially non-weight-bearing activities such as biking and swimming—are very useful in helping the runner come back from an injury, because they both help gradually improve one's fitness level and help prevent further injury. Chapter 5 lists guidelines for using alternative aerobic exercises to help you come back from injury.

PREVENTING INJURY

The use of alternative training can help prevent injury. Many aerobic exercises involve key muscle groups not sufficiently developed with a running program. Biking, for example, helps strengthen the quadriceps and thus assists in preventing knee injuries. The following chapters detail how various alternative exercises specifically assist in strengthening and stretching your musculoskeletal system and thus aid you as a runner seeking both protection from injury and increased performance. The following key muscle areas are developed with alternative aerobic exercises:

- Ankles: Swimming
- Shins: Biking (with toe clips)
- Quadriceps: Biking, race walking, cross-country skiing, rowing, swimming
- Upper body: Swimming, race walking, cross-country skiing, rowing, weight lifting
- Low back: Swimming
- Hip: Biking
- Buttocks: Race walking, cross-country skiing, rowing, swimming
- Abdomninals: Race walking, cross-country skiing, rowing

Biking, swimming, or walking after a hard workout or race helps the runner relax and recover—and prevent injury. These alternative exercises can be used in the evening and for the days after a marathon—instead of running—to ease sore muscles back into running shape. Swimming is particularly good for relaxation and postrace recovery because it provides aerobic work without the trauma of weight-bearing exercise. The water also has a massaging effect on tired muscles.

Maintaining a high level of aerobic fitness is important to the competitive runner. Aerobic benefits similar to those of running can be obtained with the use of alternative exercises. These activities can also be used to *supplement* running in order to prevent injury. Many runners would break down physically or mentally if they tried to increase their mileage beyond a certain level, especially when marathon training. These runners can enhance their training by adding alternative aerobic work to their schedule instead of spending more time pounding the roads. For example, you could add swimming or biking for 30 minutes three times a week—instead of adding another 10 miles a week of running—to increase your aerobic fitness without increasing your risk of injury.

CHOOSING AN ALTERNATIVE EXERCISE

• *Is it safe?* Check with your doctor *before* selecting any activity. Select one that will not aggravate an injury. You may wish to choose an exercise that will strengthen muscles whose weakness contributed to the injury. For example, knee pain may be alleviated by biking, which strengthens the quadriceps. The best activity maintains aerobic fitness and exercises any injured part. Slow, rhythmic movement promotes circulation, which allows for faster healing. Avoid sudden, jarring activity when injured.

According to Dr. Gabe Mirkin, in an article in *The Runner*: "Generally, the goal of any alternative sport is to retain as much endurance and strength as possible during your layoff from running without stressing your injured part. During running the greatest forces are put on your lower leg, which is why lower-leg injuries are so common among runners. Bike riding is the best alternative sport for runners with such injuries because it takes stress off the muscles of the lower leg and puts the greatest force on your hips and knees. Runners who have upper-leg injuries will find, conversely, that sports such as swimming, walking, or walking or jogging through water, which puts very little stress on your upper leg muscles, will be most beneficial to them."

• *Does it fit your schedule?* Some activities, such as walking or biking, may require twice the time devoted to running. Can you spare that? Whatever exercise you add, consider the total cost in time: swimming, for example, takes not merely time in the pool, but also time getting to and from the pool. Cross-country skiing may require traveling to the park or country—and waiting for good snow. Whatever you select, fit it to the amount of time you have allotted to exercise and the facilities and equipment available. In short, fit the exercise to where you plan to work out and how much time you have available.

• *What are your skills?* You can't jump rope without tripping, master the technique of cross-country skiing, stay afloat, or pedal very well? Fit the exercise to your skills. You need to be good enough at the activity to get in a good workout.

• *Who are you?* Do you hate the cold? Love the outdoors? Despise smelly gyms? Do pools turn you off? You will need to choose an activity that suits your personality.

TRAINING GUIDELINES FOR ALTERNATIVE AEROBIC EXERCISE

Don't just jump into an alternative exercise. You must plan your nonrunning exercise as carefully as you plan your program of running. Here are some guidelines for adding exercise to your running schedule:

• Ease into the activity. Treat your new exercise just as you did running during your first few months: Don't overdo it. Too much will be worse than too little. Because your cardiovascular system is in great shape from running, you will think that you can do more of your new activity than a conservative amount. But, because different muscles will be used or the same ones in different ways, your body will be very sore the next day if you don't start your new activity gradually. Don't cause an injury by foolishness. Begin the new exercise slowly, and do it every other day, alternating with running, if possible.

• Training principles that apply to running also apply to your alternative activity—especially the principles of alternating hard and easy days and training without overstraining.

• Perform your new exercise at an equivalent training heart rate, or perceived exertion, to that of running.

• When comparing the value of your alternative exercise to running, count the minutes you exercise in your training heart rate range. For example, swimming for one hour within your training heart rate range would be approximately equivalent to the mileage you would normally run in an hour (8 miles at a 7:30 per mile pace, for instance). This exercise is called the "running equivalent." If your exercise is less demanding than running, go longer. The rule of thumb is: If you can't reach your training heart rate, exercise at least twice as long (in terms of time) as you would have if you were running.

Your training heart rate range for aerobic exercise is 70 to 85 percent of your estimated maximum heart rate. Calculate your maximum heart rate by subtracting your age from the number 220. Here is a chart to save you the math:

TRAINING HEART RATE RANGE FOR AEROBIC EXERCISE

Age	70%	85%
20–25	140	167
26–30	134	163
31–35	131	159
36–40	127	155
41–45	124	150
46–50	120	146
51–55	117	142
56–60	113	138
61–65	110	133
66–70	106	129

Note: These pulse rates are based on a predicted maximum, and yours may not precisely correspond. The key for alternative aerobic training is to exercise at the same perceived exertion level as when running.

• If new techniques are required, take lessons (for example, in cross-country skiing).

• Whatever you select as an alternative exercise for a change of pace, continue to run a few times each week to keep your "running legs." This will ease the transition when you return to running full-time.

• If you select an alternative exercise to increase your aerobic fitness base and prevent injury, don't overdo it. You should not exceed approximately 25 percent of your total training equivalency doing alternative exercise. Thus, if you are running 60 miles a week at about a 7:30 per mile pace (8 miles per hour), don't do more than the equivalent of an additional 20 miles a week (such as 2–3 hours a week of vigorous swimming in your training heart rate range) in another activity. Don't think you are running 80-mile weeks—it's not quite the same.

• If you wish to cut back your running to rest, to baby an injury, or just for a change of pace, and wish to maintain approximately the same level of aerobic fitness with supplemental exercise, try to cut back no more than one-third of your running time. The runner doing 60 miles a week should cut back no more than 20 miles of running—to no fewer than 40 miles a week—and replace them with approximately 2–3 hours a week of alternative activity in his or her training heart rate range.

You may be able to use alternative training to simulate the cardiovascular value of running in an effort to prevent injury and increase fitness, but you should be aware that no activity uses the same specific muscle groups: You still have to get out there and pack in the miles. Hour for hour, running is the best training for the runner. Biking, swimming, race walking, and cross-country skiing are the best alternative aerobic choices for the runner. But in these, and all alternative exercises, you must keep your intensity up, not cheat, and work hard. Because running forces you to pick up your body weight and push it, it is the hardest activity to cheat at. Also, to give yourself a broader range of activities and benefits, you may want to combine alternatives: biking and weight training, for example, provide good overall workouts for the upper body, legs, and cardiovascular system.

SUCCESS STORIES

Robin Ladas is an excellent example of someone who maintained vigorous training despite not being able to run because of injury. On 70 miles a week of running, including hard speed work with her Atalanta teammates, she was able to place third in the 1980

Avon Half-Marathon in Central Park—winning an all-expense-paid trip to the 1981 Avon International Women's Marathon in Ottawa, Canada.

In the spring and summer of 1981, as she hoped to build up for her first marathon, she was forced to decrease her running because of a chronic knee problem. At one point, only a month before the marathon, she was unable to run for eighteen consecutive days. But she didn't give up! She continued to exercise by swimming and pedaling an indoor bike. She simulated her team speed workouts with challenging sessions on the bike or in the pool. She was forced to stand up on her bike and pedal against the full resistance of the brake in order to drive her body into oxygen debt. Robin even swam with flippers flexed and bent at right angles, using only her arms against the dragging action for 400 strokes (yes, she counted them).

Before the August marathon she was able to get in one week of 45 miles of running and then a tapering week of 30 miles. On race day, she started conservatively in very hot, humid weather and ran a steady pace. Her secret strength training paid off as she moved up over 100 places in the last half of the race and just missed by one place the silver necklace given to the top 30. Robin ran an incredible first marathon of 2:58:15. She proved that if you *have to* train for a big race—but can't run—it is possible to succeed. But you need to plan carefully and be very dedicated and determined.

Eric Ryan took up alternative forms of exercise when he couldn't run because of injury after he completed the 1980 New York Marathon in 2:51. He had trained the traditional way—60 miles a week, long runs, and speed work. Once injured, he joined his injured wife for long bike rides and weight training. Eventually, he could run again, but couldn't train hard for the 1981 New York Marathon. So he ran 20 miles a week, biked 80–100 miles a week, and did vigorous weight training three times a week. He did his "long runs" on an outdoor bike and found that 100-milers were about equal to 22–25 mile runs in terms of cardiovascular value. His speed work was on an indoor bike. A week before the marathon he put in one last mental and physical preparation workout. For 1½ hours he pushed hard, nonstop, rotating among lowweight, high-repetition work with Nautilus equipment, the stationary bike, rope skipping, and running in place. After that, he was mentally ready.

Eric felt much stronger in the upper body and quads but a little short on endurance going into the race. He ran the marathon in the same time he had the year before, on a third of the mileage. It's interesting that his body weight going into the 1980 event was 142 pounds and body fat 7.9 percent. A year later, using alternative training, he weighed 12 pounds more, but his body fat percentage was almost the same. Thus he weighed more, but was more solid, especially in the upper body and legs.

Kass Young had been a runner in high school and college, but became a rower when she was working on her doctorate degree at Oxford University. In fact, she was good enough to compete for the women's crew team. After returning to New York City in 1980, she resumed her running and joined Bob Glover's Atalanta team. Her progress was steady, and she ran the September 1981 Avon Half-Marathon in a strong 1:24. Shortly thereafter, she developed chronic foot and ankle problems and was forced to stop running completely.

For the next six months Kass swam about 30 minutes a day, five times a week to maintain aerobic fitness. She hated it and finally—in desperation—bought an indoor rowing machine. She gradually returned to rowing and eased out of swimming. For nine months she ran an easy 8–10 minutes each morning, building up to 20 minutes—the limit for her injury—and then rowed for a brisk 30 minutes. She did anaerobic speed work twice a week using these basic workouts, patterned after her crew sessions at Oxford:

1. Row hard for 1 minute, easy for 1 minute. Repeat for a total of five to six times.
2. Row a pyramid: Hard 1 minute, easy 1 minute; hard 2 minutes, easy 2 minutes; hard 3 minutes, easy 3 minutes; hard 2 minutes, easy 2 minutes; hard 1 minute, easy 1 minute.
3. Row hard 5 minutes, easy 5 minutes. Repeat for a total of three to four times.
4. Do speed bursts—similar to fartleks—over 20 minutes.

By the winter of 1982, Kass was spending 45–60 minutes each day doing the two activities. She couldn't run for longer than 30 minutes, but she also couldn't row much longer than that. The major muscle groups are exercised so powerfully on the rowing machine that she would tire before her cardiovascular system wore down. Thus, to get in more than 30 minutes of aerobic work, she combined it with 30 minutes of running.

In January 1983 Kass returned to the vigorous Atalanta speed workouts. Her program for the next four months consisted of

- 20–25 miles per week of running, including one team speed session
- 30–35 minutes of rowing, six days per week (she didn't row the day she ran speed workouts) for a "running equivalent" of 20–25 miles per week, including one rowing speed session
- A total running equivalent of 40–50 miles per week with two speed sessions

In May 1983 she ran her first race in over a year and a half. She won a women's only 5-mile race in Central Park with a personal record of 30:18.

Rowing is an excellent alternative training exercise that builds aerobic endurance, anaerobic capacity, and upper- and lower-body strength. Running and rowing complement each other well. Rowing exercises many of the same muscles that are used in running, plus muscles that are not used: quadriceps, abdominals, buttocks, and upper body. We do not include a chapter on rowing in this book, but it certainly should be considered as an aerobic alternative for the injured runner.

8 BIKING

Biking is an excellent alternative exercise for the runner. Here are some of its benefits:

Increases Aerobic Endurance. According to aerobics guru Dr. Kenneth Cooper, biking is "a good match for running. The aerobic benefits—the training effect—to the internal organs are identical with those of running." The key is to keep your heart rate up in your training range—approximately at the same level as when running—for the same period of time as when running. Thus, a 30-minute run and a 30-minute bike ride are approximately of equal value to your cardiovascular conditioning if both are done at an equivalent training heart rate.

Burns Calories. Biking burns approximately 700 calories per hour at a brisk pace of 15 miles per hour. Running burns approximately 800 calories per hour at a brisk running pace of 7½ minutes per mile.

Balances Muscle Development. Biking also complements the muscular demands of running. Runners develop strong hamstring muscles, but running largely neglects the opposing quadriceps, leaving the runner prone to knee injuries. Dr. Edward Colt, an avid runner and biker, treats many of New York City's injured runners. He likes biking because it "particularly strengthens the quadricep (upper thigh) muscles and (if toe clips are used) the anterior shin muscles (minimizing shin splints). These two muscle groups are vulnerable in runners and they are not really strengthened by running. The action of biking on the quadriceps muscle stabilizes the knee joint and eases virtually all knee pains. Biking relaxes the calf and hamstring muscles and is excellent therapy for tightening, strains or tears in these two muscle groups." Strengthening the quads through biking will also help the runner fight fatigue when he or she must use these muscles to pick up the knees while racing up hills or during the late stages of a marathon.

Improves Flexibility. According to Sally Edwards, a national-class triathlon athlete, biking increases flexibility in the hip and knee joints: "The impact running has on the joints tends to tighten the connective tissue that surrounds them. Cycling, on the other hand, tends to stretch the connective tissue because in the cycling motion, the knee almost fully extends while supporting very little body weight. Also, the greater range of motion in cycling should produce greater flexibility."

Helps Rehabilitate Injuries. Biking is especially good for runners with injuries requiring non-weight-bearing exercise, such as stress fractures, or those with leg casts. Before Carl Eilenberg became mayor of Rome, New York, he was forced to use an indoor bike for exercise after breaking his leg. With a leg cast up to his hip, Carl worked out on his indoor bike. He built up to 30–60 minutes daily, pumping with his good leg and hanging the cast off to one side. Later, in a half-cast up to his knee, he could pedal with both legs. By the time he returned to running, Carl was more fit than before he was injured.

Aids Recovery from Hard Work. In the days following a tough race or hard speed workout, biking can help you recover properly. It forces blood into the aching legs and removes waste products, which cause stiffness, without further jarring the muscles and joints.

Serves as a Warm-up for Running. Especially on cold days, a prerun workout of 15–20 minutes on an indoor bike will warm up your stiff muscles, loosen joints, and minimize injury. You can also ride your outdoor bike a few miles to and from your workout to aid in your warm-up and cool-down.

Supplements Running Training. Biking doesn't have to be used only as an alternative exercise when you can't run because of an injury. It can also be used to supplement your training, both to improve fitness and prevent injury. In addition to the benefits listed above, biking can greatly relieve the mental and physical stresses of the runner's training program. Dr. Alex Ratelle, a national-class masters champion and 2:30 marathoner at the age of fifty-seven, is an outspoken promoter of the benefits of biking to supplement running. Of course, since he lives and trains in Minnesota, where the winter temperatures frequently go way below zero, he is often forced indoors to look for alternatives to running. Ratelle commented in an interview in *The Runner*, "If I tried to get all my calorie burning and cardiovascular conditioning from running I'd be constantly injured. And there are times when I'm just mentally sick of running. During those times I can ride the bike, and soothe my conscience because I didn't miss my workouts."

INDOORS VERSUS OUTDOORS

One advantage of biking is that it can be done indoors on a stationary bike or outdoors. On an indoor bike, you can regulate your heart rate by adjusting the speed and resistance of the bike, as well as monitor your heart rate to ensure proper training. With outdoor biking, you must constantly push hard to keep your pulse up in the training range. The more fit you are, the faster you need to pedal. You must search for biking paths or country roads that are free of traffic lights, cars, pedestrians, and other interruptions that will lower the quality of your workout. It is much easier to control your workout on an indoor bike. You don't have to slow down for turns or people; you don't have steep uphills, which dramatically increase your pulse above your training range, or long downhills, where you tend to coast and drop your pulse below your training range. On an indoor bike you can easily measure your pulse and adjust the pace by either increasing or decreasing the speed you are pedaling or the resistance of the brake.

HOW FAST, HOW FAR, HOW LONG: BIKING VERSUS RUNNING

To match your running workout with equivalent biking exercise, you'll have to pedal *about twice as fast, for a greater distance, for at least the same period of time.* Each runner's equivalent work load as a biker will be influenced by such factors as whether you are biking indoors or outdoors; the bike; if outdoors, the weather; your biking skill and fitness level; and the terrain.

Speed. Generally, a pace slower than 10 miles per hour will not be aerobically beneficial, whereas faster than 20 miles per hour is racing speed and will bring about oxygen debt and rapid fatigue. The average runner-biker should train at 12–15 miles per hour. This speed would keep his or her heart rate in the 70 to 85 percent of maximum range and bring about a perceived exertion similar to that of the average daily run.

Distance. Because you'll be traveling faster on a bike than while running, you will be covering a greater distance. Generally, 3–5 miles of biking is the training equivalent of 1 mile of running.

Time. If you are able to keep your pulse in your training range, the time involved in equivalent training with biking is the same as running; thus, you can replace running aerobically minute for minute with biking. This is easier to do on an indoor bike, where you can control the environment and adjust the resistance of the bike to maintain steady effort. The longer you bike outdoors, and the less skilled you are as a biker or the less fit you are, the harder it is to keep your pulse up in your training range. If you fall below 70 percent of your maximum heart rate (your minimum target), you will need to bike for a longer time than you would run to get an equivalent aerobic workout—one and a half to two times as long.

In an interesting experiment, Vince McDonald and Mike Cleary raced the 6-mile loop of New York City's Central Park. A few years earlier they had been of equal running ability, but McDonald had been forced to give up running by a nagging back injury. Instead, he became a fine competitive cyclist, while Cleary went on to become a top local marathoner, with a time of 2:23. The race was two loops of biking versus one of running. Incredibly, they finished at exactly the same time. A skilled biker racing for short distances can cover twice the distance of a runner over a period of 30 minutes to an hour. If you are an average runner, you would bike 3–4 miles to reach the training equivalent of running for 1 mile. However, you would have to bike 5–6 miles or more for each mile of running if you bike at a slow pace, go for a long bike ride, or are unskilled as a biker.

GUIDELINES FOR BIKERS

Novice bikers, just like first-time runners, make errors in training and technique that are obstacles to improvement and causes of injury.

Here are some guidelines to help you avoid those pitfalls:

• Ease into your biking mileage, just as you did with your running. Start with rides of 20–30 minutes, and gradually increase to the equivalent time of your running. Don't ride for more than an hour at once until your legs, buttocks, and upper body have adjusted to the new strains and stresses. You will discover that your legs will fatigue and your upper body, hands, and neck— along with your fanny—will become uncomfortable long before your heart and lungs give out.

• You can safely use running shoes to pedal with, but if you plan to start doing long rides or racing you should consider special biking shoes, which have less flexible soles to keep your feet from flexing and overworking. If you wear orthotics in your running shoes, especially a metatarsal correction or support, wear them in your biking shoes as well. The ball of the foot, pushing on the pedal, receives a lot of stress.

• Your knees will also benefit from biking if you avoid several possible causes of knee pain. Knee pain can be caused by setting a bicycle seat at an improper height. The seat is at the proper height if your knee is only slightly bent at extension. Knee pain can also occur as a result of pedaling too hard in high gear. Lower your gear, and learn to use toe clips to increase your power and efficiency. Toe clips hold the front part of your feet on the pedals to give you power through the full range of motion, both pushing and pulling. They also increase the involvement of the quadricep muscles and the muscles in the front of your shins.

In an article on biking that appeared in *Runner's World*, Sally Edwards listed five common errors of new bikers:

"1. *Spinning too slowly in too high a gear.* This is inefficient and can put too much stress on leg muscles. Try to spin in a gear that is aerobically comfortable (remember the "talk test" in running?) at a rate of 60–70 rpm.

2. *Riding too fast too soon.* Again, remember what it was like when you first began to run—there was a temptation to run too fast. This happens to riders as well. Slow down and ride longer.

3. *Having an improperly set-up bicycle.* Adjust your bike to fit you for power, safety and comfort.

4. *Riding inefficiently.* Try to develop a smooth pedaling technique and try to keep your body compact, thereby minimizing wind resistance.

5. *Not being cautious enough.* When you're riding a bicycle, you're often going at speeds that can spell disaster or death in case of a mishap. Wear a helmet and other

proper safety gear—reflectors, light, visible clothing, gloves and so on. *Ride defensively*—don't run yellow or red lights at intersections, and pay attention to your greatest nemesis, the automobile."

SAMPLE TRAINING PROGRAM

Follow a training program using the same principles as for running. You may wish to add long rides or speed work to your biking program, especially if you can't train by running and are preparing for a key race. First develop a base of 30–60 minutes of steady biking, and then ease into your speed work. Don't forget to take rest days before and after speed days and long rides. As for running, thoroughly warm up with stretching and easy biking and then reverse the procedure for the cool-down.

Sample Speed Workouts on a Bike

Outdoors:
1. Pedal very hard for 20–30 minutes, at approximately 85 percent of your maximum heart rate.
2. Pedal very hard for 3–8 minutes, then pedal at a moderate pace for 2 minutes. Do six to eight sets. This simulates track workouts of ½–1 mile.
3. Push hard uphill for 3–5 minutes, and return downhill. Repeat six to eight times.

Indoors:
1. Same as 1 and 2 above.
2. Pedal very hard (almost all-out) against very strong resistance for 30 seconds, then bike easy for 15–30 seconds. Repeat for six to ten sets. This simulates doing short sprints on a track or running up short, steep hills.

SUCCESS STORIES

Richard Traum lost his right leg above the knee as a result of a freak accident. In 1975, as his weight and blood pressure were rapidly increasing, he decided to start running and enrolled in one of Bob Glover's programs. He went on to complete the New York Marathon six times, running on an artificial leg. But in 1978 he wasn't able to run the marathon because of problems with his only knee. In fact, he hardly ran at all that year. Dick tried biking indoors but found it boring. Eventually, he started indoor biking at Glover's insistence for 40 minutes at a time three times a week just to maintain minimal fitness.

In late May 1979 Dick decided that he would start training for the marathon, and with Glover's help he laid out a unique plan. They determined that he would train for the marathon on the bike and do a minimal amount of running, and then on race day he would take his time, alternating running and walking; he would not attempt to beat his personal record of 6:44, set in 1977. So Dick pedaled away—pushing with his good leg on one pedal and a crutch on the other.

He built up to a three day a week training routine: one day of running up to 5 miles, one day of indoor biking for 2 hours, and one of 4 hours. Often he would do "pickups" for 2–3 minutes on the bike to relieve boredom. He played with the height and angle of the seat to relieve his biggest problem—"fanny fatigue"—and noticed that TV programs were much better than a few years ago.

Dick ran a 5-mile race and a 20-kilometer race (his longest run) to test his knee, and, on a very hot day, he "negotiated" the New York Marathon course in 8:04. Starting in 1980 he did a little biking and a little running to keep in shape until the summer of 1981. Then he added a few longer bike rides in preparation for another marathon effort. His big one was 110 kilometers while watching TV from 6:00 to 11:30 p.m. on a Saturday night. Every hour he would get off to change his shirt and go to the bathroom. Despite a diagnosed arthritic knee, he completed the 1981 New York Marathon in 7:21. In the fall of 1982, Dick encouraged Glover to cofound the Achilles Track Club, a running club for the physically disabled. This group of runners compete in wheelchairs, on crutches, with canes, with artificial legs, and so on and prove that minor injuries shouldn't be obstacles to the able-bodied runner.

Only nine weeks before the 1982 New York Marathon, Californian Lou Kwiker suffered an injury as a result of a biking accident. Determined to compete in his first marathon, he followed this successful program:

After receiving emergency treatment at the hospital, he went home and stayed in bed for four days. Following the injury, his leg increased in circumference by 5 full inches because of swelling. For these first days he iced the leg constantly and then started heat treatments. A week after the injury he started to exercise the leg gently in a whirlpool. Three days later he walked for the first time and began to bike easily for 20 minutes at a time. A week later he started a program of running alternated with outdoor biking, gradually increasing his running.

Lou notes, "In summary, during the 9 weeks before the marathon I ran a total of 182 miles, or roughly 20 miles a week. In addition, I biked 475 miles, or 190 running mile equivalents, for an average of about 21 miles a week. Therefore my combined running and biking mileage averaged 41 miles a week after the injury.

"I feel that I would have been unable to run the marathon without the biking exercise. My leg would not have been able to take more running than I actually gave to it and the biking provided me with the necessary speedwork and the aerobic effort that was necessary to run decently." He finished in 3:42:55.

The following year, in consultation with Glover, Lou devised a plan to improve his time: He would run 50 miles a week and add another 20 miles a week with "biking equivalents" to give him a 70 mile a week basis—a mileage level that he would not be able to handle with just running. He completed the 1983 New York Marathon in 3:29:54.

As a high-school senior in upstate New York, Cindi Girard placed third in the 2-mile at the state track meet. As a seventeen-year-old college freshman she set an American record for age nineteen and under with a 1:19:43 half-marathon in Central Park. Shortly thereafter she quit running for over three years. In April 1983— 25 pounds overweight—she started running again and cautiously returned to racing. In August she joined Atalanta and by October ran a 34:41 10-kilometer. Realizing the risk of injury from doing too much too soon, she trained to fulfill a dream—qualifying for the Olympic trials. Following a conservative training schedule, she built up her endurance and strength and qualified in her *first* marathon with a 2:49:12 in Jacksonville in January 1984.

Coming off the race, however, she was very tight in her legs and hips. Glover sent her to a physical therapist to prevent an injury from destroying her promising running career. Besides physical therapy treatment, Cindi was given a program of stretching and strengthening exercises to improve her flexibility and balance muscular strength. Glover helped her work out a biking program, initially to replace her running and later to supplement it. She started riding an indoor bike each morning for 40 minutes (about equal to a 5-mile run) and doing a 5-mile run each evening. This gave her the aerobic equivalent of 60–70 miles a week of running, but lessened the shock on her legs and hips. Gradually she worked up to 60 miles a week of running, but continued to bike several times a week to increase her aerobic endurance. She also biked instead of running the day after her weekly team speed workout on the road or track and any day when slippery footing caused by snow or ice could aggravate her injury. Further, Cindi did two speed workouts per week on the bike in addition to her hard session of running as she sharpened for racing. If she had attempted to run hard more often she would have been very prone to injury. Because her long runs aggravated the condition, she instead biked for 30 minutes before and after runs of 10–15 miles to replace 20-mile long runs. Following this routine Cindi prevented a major injury and actually became a more balanced and efficient runner because the biking strengthened her quadriceps while her stretching program improved flexibility in the backs of her legs and hips. She also didn't feel as tired as she had when she "burned out" as a college freshman on a program of over 80 miles of running each week. In the June 1984 L'eggs Mini Marathon in New York, she placed fourteenth in a record field of over 7,000 women. Cindi enthusiastically promotes the use of an indoor bike to prevent injury and improve performance.

FOR MORE INFORMATION

Check with your local bike specialty shop or a local biking club for assistance with such details as proper technique, safety and training guidelines, and proper choice and use of equipment. The following sources are also recommended.

Books

Anybody's Bike Book by
Tom Cuthbertson
(Berkeley, CA: Ten Speed Press, 1979).

Everybody's Book of Bicycle Riding by Tom Lieb
(Emmaus, PA: Rodale Press, 1981).

Get Fit with Bicycling
(Emmaus, PA: Bicycling Magazine, 1979).

The Complete Book of Bicycling by Eugene A. Sloane
(New York, NY: Simon & Schuster, 1974).

Magazine

Bicycling Magazine
Rodale Press, Emmaus, PA   18049

Organizations

American Bicycling Association
P.O. Box 718
Chandler, AZ   85224

Bicycle Institute of America
122 East Forty-second Street
New York, NY   10017

League of American Wheelmen
Box 988
Baltimore, MD   21203

United States Cycling Federation
680 Rutland Avenue
Teaneck, NJ   07666

9 SWIMMING

Dr. Kenneth Cooper, author of several books on aerobics, ranks the four most effective aerobic activities in this order: cross-country skiing, swimming, running, and biking. Cooper says, "As the second most effective aerobic exercise, swimming involves all of the major muscles of the body, and as a result, it gives you more of a total conditioning effect than many other sports. Also, swimmers tend to have fewer problems with injuries than runners because the buoyancy of the water helps reduce excessive pressure on the joints and bones." Gordon Stewart, author of *Every Body's Fitness Book*, proclaims, "The water has something for everyone. It's an ideal medium for those with back problems, arthritis, and other joint disorders. Physiotherapists have long used it for retraining and rehabilitation from injury, illness, and accident. For fitness, swimming brings a balanced development—upper and lower body strength and suppleness that no other single activity can match."

Here are some of the benefits of swimming:

Increases Aerobic Endurance. Dr. Cooper ranks swimming as having nearly the same aerobic benefits as running and biking. Once again, a 30-minute swim is equal to a 30-minute run if you keep your heart in the training range. Jane Katz, author of *Swimming for Total Fitness*, observes, "Swimming has this added effect: When your body is horizontal and immersed in water, your heart is actually larger than when you're vertical on dry land and it has to pump against gravity. As a result, between 10 and 20 percent more blood is pumped with each heart contraction. This effect gives you the potential to work harder and longer than you ever could on land."

Burns Calories. Swimming burns approximately 600 calories per hour, depending on your stroke, speed, and skill as a swimmer.

Balances Muscle Development. Running does little for your upper body, whereas swimming exercises the entire body—arms, shoulders, abdominals, hips, legs, and ankles.

Improves Flexibility. According to Katz, "Swimming's long, sinuous motions, along with the increased range of movement that your body has in the water, actually elongates your muscles while strengthening them. Swimming will help loosen you up—both in the water and after you're out."

Helps Rehabilitate Injuries. Swimming is probably the least stressful alternative exercise, and therefore ideal after injury. Water movement around the injured area has therapeutic benefits, and swimming seems to ensure more blood supply to injured areas and improve the possibility of quick recovery. Besides swimming to keep in shape and decrease recovery time, you can also run in shallow water, which minimizes stress to the legs; run using a flotation device; or use hydrotherapy—active or passive movements while partially or completely submerged in warm water.

According to physical therapist Robert Kropf, "hydrotherapy offers many advantages to the runner, and one of the most important is providing an isokinetic exercise environment. When we push our muscles against a resistance that is constant in speed, thereby using the full strength of muscles through their full range of movement, we are exercising in an isokinetic fashion. Most experts agree that isokinetic exercise is the best way to rehabilitate athletes. The basic idea behind this is that we want to exercise muscles in a manner that is most similar in speed and type to the activity the athlete wishes to return to. Walking, jogging, and running in the pool are fantastic ways to rehabilitate a runner. The pool provides resistance at all speeds of participation (isokinetics), and the runner is exercising in a similar manner to the activity to which he or she wants to return."

Aids Recovery from Hard Work. Swimming is also relaxing. Pete Schuder, coauthor of *The Competitive Runner's Handbook*, found that swimming helped him relax and sleep better after "running himself into the ground" in tough speed workouts. Swimming also helps stretch out tired muscles, thus minimizing injury. Runners should consider using a 20–30 minute swim to cool down after a hard workout instead of jogging for a few more miles and adding more pounding on stiff muscles. Swimming is especially valuable when recovering from a marathon.

Enhances Breathing and Rhythm. When swimming you must really concentrate on your breathing. The result is that you learn to inhale and exhale more completely and more rhythmically. This control of your breathing carries over into your running and helps you control the "panic breathing" that may occur in races. There is some evidence that because you have to restrict your breathing when swimming with your head under water you improve your respiratory system's ability to diffuse oxygen. Patty Lee Parmalee, Atalanta's national-class masters runner, maintains that swimming increases the runner's gracefulness and thus enhances running style. While in Cuba for a month in 1983 she was forced to do most of her New York Marathon build-up training by swimming in the ocean. She felt that the fluidity of swimming made her more conscious of good running style when she returned to land. When she came back to running she perceived "sort of a smoother, more coordinated feeling in my arms, and more strength in the triceps area."

Cools the Body. Because while swimming your body is completely surrounded by water, which has a cooling effect, you can exercise with no fear of overheating—no matter how hot it is outside. Thus, the runner may use swimming as an alternative workout to escape extreme heat. Also, because of the water's rapid dissipation of heat generated through exercise, you fatigue less quickly and recover more quickly than when exercising in the medium of air.

Supplements Running Training. National-class masters runner Hal Higdon emphasized in an article in *The Runner* that rehabilitation after an injury is the main reason runners swim. . . . But a second area, largely unexplored by coaches, is to use swimming as a supplement to running. A runner capable of running only a certain number of miles a week because of the trauma associated with 1,000 foot-steps a mile may be able to improve his physical capacity by swimming." In fact, Brooks Johnson, 1984 U.S. women's Olympic track coach and track coach at Stanford University, has his national powerhouse women's college distance running squad swim several mornings a week to supplement their running. He feels "the conditioning you get from swimming is superior to that you get from running" because swimming reduces the wear and tear on the body while still improving aerobic fitness. Thus, he uses swimming to replace the traditional morning run in the typical two run a day schedule used by top high-mileage runners.

DISADVANTAGES OF SWIMMING

• Most runners are impatient people accustomed to running in interesting scenery and chatting with others on the run. An athlete has to be patient and disciplined to train in the limited atmosphere of swimming. A 30-minute swim for a runner may seem to last twice as long as an hour's run. It may help to break up the swim with different strokes per lap, or to alternate a hard swim with a brief rest rather than swimming one monotonous lap after another. Another way to avoid boredom is to swim in a pond, lake, stream, or the ocean. The change in scenery can be inspiring even for a runner. Swimming in ocean or lake waves can also add fun to the workout. Be sure to swim with a partner or, when alone, in shallow water or close to the shore.

• According to Michael Houston, an exercise physiologist at the University of Waterloo in Ontario, athletes who have used swimming as an alternative activity maintain aerobic fitness, but their muscular fitness decreases. Swimming improves upper-body strength, but it doesn't do much for the lower-body muscles that are specific to running. In an interview with Hal Higdon for *The Runner*, Nike exercise physiologist Jack Daniels warned that "a runner may come out of the pool in good cardiovascular shape, and aggravate his injury, or cause a new one, by going too hard too fast. It may be an advantage to be equally out of shape in all areas, circulatory and muscular, because you won't be able to push yourself into another injury."

There are three ways to prevent injury in this case: (1) maintain a minimal amount of running to keep the running-specific muscles in shape; (2) add weight training to work the neglected muscles; (3) exercise the running-specific muscles by impersonating a runner in the water: "running" upright in deep water using a flotation device.

• When you are swimming, it is more difficult to get your heart rate up into your training range because your body is horizontal. You have to work really hard to exercise properly, not just float along in the water. Conversely, unskilled swimmers may find it easy to get their heart rate up, but hard to swim for very long because their "swimming muscles"—unconditioned and inefficient—will tire before they can complete a workout equivalent to a running session.

• Finding an uncrowded pool is difficult. It may also be expensive.

• Swimming prevents you from sweating or getting hot. Returning to racing from this totally different medium can require acclimatization.

HOW FAST, HOW FAR, HOW LONG: SWIMMING VERSUS RUNNING

You'll swim at a slower pace, for a shorter distance, but for at least the same amount of time to get a workout equivalent to running. Each runner's equivalent work load as a swimmer will be influenced by such factors as fitness level, skill as a swimmer, type of stroke used, length of pool, and whether the pool is crowded.

Speed. If you are an average runner, you will cover 1–2 miles per hour (compared to 6–8 miles per hour running)—depending on your skill and the distance you are swimming. An excellent swimmer may cover a mile in 30 minutes, a good swimmer in 40–50 minutes, and a less skilled, less conditioned swimmer in 50–60 minutes. Because of the nature of swimming, the training heart rate range is lowered from 70 to 85 percent for runners to 60 to 85 percent for swimmers. Unless you are unskilled and struggling, or skilled and pushing very hard, your training pulse may be about 10 beats per minute less for the perceived effort because you are lying horizontally and buoyant in the water and your body has less resistance. Also, the water acts as a coolant, holding down both heart rate and temperature.

Distance. Swimming ¼–⅕ mile is about the same as running 1 mile. Thus, a mile of swimming is roughly equivalent to 4–5 miles of running.

Time. Runners insist on counting mileage. Swimmers, however, swim for time rather than count laps. If you are able to keep your pulse in your training heart rate range (60–85% of it for swimming), the time involved in equivalent training is the same as running. Thus, it is possible to substitute running aerobically minute for minute with swimming. If you fall below 60 percent of your maximum heart rate, you will need to swim for longer than you usually run to get an equivalent aerobic workout—one and a half to two times as long.

GUIDELINES FOR SWIMMERS

When you start swimming, you must be careful to follow common-sense training guidelines. Here are some tips for swimmer-runners:

• Start your workout by stretching on land, then do some easy laps to warm up. After your workout swim easy laps for 3–5 minutes to cool down.

• The first goal as a beginner is to build up to swimming 1 mile, then up to your approximately daily average as a runner. One mile is 72 laps of a 25-meter pool. At first, swim only 20–30 minutes; then gradually increase the time. It will take you about 40–60 minutes of swimming to reach your 1-mile goal.

• Consider swimming intervals of 2–10 minutes at a fairly brisk pace, with rest breaks of 10–40 seconds. Try this pyramid workout: Swim 1 lap, rest; swim 2 laps, rest; swim 3 laps, rest; swim 2 laps, rest; swim 1 lap, rest. This workout fights boredom, keeps you from quitting, and rests your upper-body muscles. It will also allow you to swim fast enough to keep your heart rate up. This may be the most efficient way to train. Also, you can use the runner's fartlek workout: Swim alternating laps hard and easy.

• Stay relaxed as you swim, and breathe rhythmically. Breathe in and out using both your mouth and nose.

• Take Jane Katz's advice: "The first thing people have to know is how to breathe as they swim. Most people overkick, using the big muscles of their legs too much, and they build up an oxygen debt. Their arms should be 70 percent of the stroke."

• For variety, and for a more balanced exercise program, you may choose to rotate strokes for part of your swim. The major strokes are freestyle, backstroke, breaststroke, sidestroke, and butterfly. All exercise most of your major muscles and joints, but certain strokes are better than others for particular muscle groups.

Freestyle. According to Sally Edwards, "the freestyle is not only the most efficient stroke in swimming, it's also the stroke that works best for your body. Don't chop at the water; concentrate on making long, graceful strokes and try to get as much distance as possible from each one. . . . Swim with your arms, using your legs for balance. 'Pull' on the water and try to bring your arms in and out of the water with as small a splash as possible." The chance of injury with this stroke is very small, and the flutter kick is great for relaxing tight muscles.

Backstroke. The backstroke loosens tight back muscles after long runs and races.

Breaststroke. Because it uses the whip kick, the breaststroke strengthens thigh muscles. However, this kick can cause knee problems and create a strain on your outside ankle.

Sidestroke. The sidestroke is a simple stroke used primarily for warm-up, cool-down, or recovery after harder work.

Butterfly. The butterfly is the most difficult and strenuous stroke because it has no rest cycle. It is recommended only for the fit, skilled swimmer.

GUIDELINES FOR SPEED WORK

The runner forced into the pool can continue to train competitively. Long swims, a combination of running or biking followed by a swim, can replace the long endurance run. Anaerobic speed work can be done using one of three methods: (1) alternating hard swimming laps with easy laps or rest; (2) running hard in the shallow end of the pool; (3) running hard in the deep end using a flotation device.

Follow the same training guidelines you use in running, especially alternating hard days with easy days. Here are some sample speed workouts that can be used in the pool:

Swimming
- Swim hard for 3–8 minutes, then swim easy for 2–3 minutes. Do six to eight sets. This parallels running ½–1 mile track workouts. Alberto Salazar used this type of workout combined with indoor biking to keep in shape during an eight-week layoff before qualifying for the 1980 Olympic team at 10 kilometers. His 300-yard repetitions in the pool took 4:17, which he equated in terms of time and effort with about one hard mile on the track.
- To strengthen your arms and shoulders, swim hard, using only your arms, for 2 or 3 minutes. Cross your feet and hook them.
- Swim interval sprints of 50–100 yards, with rest periods of 1–2 minutes. Do these at an effort similar to that of quarter-miles on a track. Do four to ten sets.
- Swim continuously doing fartlek bursts: swim 1 lap hard, 1 easy; 2 hard, 2 easy; and so on.
- To strengthen the quadriceps, tread water for 15–30 minutes, and concentrate on lifting the knees. Feel that you are "running in the water."

Using Flotation Devices
- Hold on to a Styrofoam board and kick hard for 1 lap of the pool. Rest as needed and repeat several times. This is particularly good for the legs.
- Wear a life jacket to "run" with your legs in the deep end of the pool. Do long runs or speed workouts for 3–8 minutes, followed by 2–3 easy minutes. Keep your body vertical in a running position, rather than horizontal in the swimming position. This allows you to mimic the running action

without the trauma of pounding the roads.

Dr. David Brody, medical director of the Marine Corps Marathon in Washington, DC, studied eight runners for an eight-week period. They followed an exact schedule of runs—speed training, easy runs, long runs—and did all their "running" in the deep end of a pool wearing life jackets. All of them improved their marathon times and suffered no foot or leg injuries despite being off the road for two months. It must be pointed out that these runners were in good shape and used this alternative training method to maintain fitness, rather than to get into marathon shape to start with. This type of training better prepares the runner's muscles for returning to competitive running than straight swimming.

Shallow Water Training
- Stand in the water up to your waist. Run widths of the pool against resistance. Build up to 30 minutes.
- Stand in water up to your thighs. Run sprints, concentrating on raising the knees.

Note: The buoyancy of the water minimizes pounding and lessens the aggravation of injury. However, for injuries such as stress fractures of the feet and plantar fasciitis, pushing off the foot—even when the shock is minimized—could cause problems. When exercising in shallow water, be careful to avoid the tendency to twist the upper body—this could cause back injury.

SAMPLE TRAINING PROGRAM

As described in Chapter 5, Angella Hearn was sidelined for several weeks and forced to do all her training in a swimming pool. After only a few days of running following her swimming program, she ran a PR of 2:50:05 in the London Marathon. Here is the program that proved successful for her.

She swam for one hour each morning before work and for one-half hour each evening after work for four full weeks and

didn't run a step. She trained six days a week using this schedule:
Mornings:

1. Four fast laps freestyle
2. Two slow laps breaststroke
3. Four laps breaststroke with flutter kick to work the leg muscles

She repeated this sequence eight to twelve times four mornings per week. Two mornings she swam for a steady hour.

Evenings: For one-half hour she treaded water, lifting her knees as if she were running and driving her arms.

As she eased back into running, she continued to do her speed work in the pool.

SUCCESS STORY

John Bell is a forty-five-year-old corporate president from Marion, Indiana. He completed his first marathon, the 1980 New York Marathon, in over 4 hours. The following two years he improved his time, but was not able to reach his potential because of injuries caused by his inability to handle high mileage and hard speed work. For the 1983 New York Marathon, his training schedule was revised to include only 50–60 miles a week of running and one speed workout per week. Instead of running a second speed workout each week and adding another 20 miles a week of running to make John strong enough to break the 3-hour barrier, he and Bob Glover substituted swimming workouts. John's success with this system is best described in his own words:

"I feel the benefit to me was an increased level of endurance and speed with no injuries to legs or ankles, which I had experienced in the previous 3 years whenever I got my total weekly mileage above the 70-mile mark, and tried to do too much speed work or hill training. Thanks to the new training system, my time has decreased as follows: the first New York Marathon I ran was in 1980 at 4:15:44, and 9,977th place. In 1981 my time was 3:44:27

and 6,954th place. In 1982 I reduced that to 3:38:55 and 6,452nd place. In 1983, with the aid of the revised method of training, combined with the swimming, I lowered my time to 2:57:53 and an overall place of 1,356. I firmly believe that without the revised training schedule and the addition of the swimming, I would not have been able to run a sub-3-hour marathon in 1983." With increased running mileage supplemented with swimming, John ran the hot 1984 New York Marathon in 2:46.

All kinds of workouts are possible for swimmers and non-swimmers in pools, oceans, lakes—even bathtubs. Rumor has it that the great Czech runner Emil Zatopek—winner of the 5-kilometer, 10-kilometer, and marathon in the 1952 Olympics—found an unusual alternative exercise when his wife was very ill and he had to remain by her side. He placed a pile of towels at the bottom of the bathtub, filled it halfway with water, and ran vigorously in place for an hour at a time.

FOR MORE INFORMATION

Check with a swimming instructor for help with proper technique and training guidelines. Following are sources for more information:

Books
Swimming for Total Fitness: A Progressive Aerobic Program by Jane Katz, Ed. D. (Garden City, NY: Dolphin Books, Doubleday, 1981).
Donna DeVarona's Hydro-Aerobics (Macmilliam, 1984).

Magazines
Swim Swim
P.O. Box 5901
Santa Monica, CA 90405
Swimmers Magazine
P.O. Box 15906
Nashville, TN 37215

Organization
Council for National Cooperation in Aquatics
220 Ashton Road
Ashton, MD 20702

10 WALKING

According to the American Heart Association, "Walking briskly—not just strolling—is the simplest and also one of the best forms of exercise." No special equipment is needed, other than a good pair of walking or running shoes, and you can walk anywhere at any time. Walking is also extremely popular. According to the President's Council on Physical Fitness and Sports, over 36 million Americans over age eighteen walk regularly for exercise. In fact, the group hike held throughout Europe, called a *volksmarch*, is growing so popular in America that it has begun to rival running events in several parts of the country for numbers of participants. The American Volksport Association stages hundreds of events around the country.

Here are some of the benefits of walking and hiking:

Increases Aerobic Endurance. According to exercise physiologist Dr. Michael Pollack, walking is of equal aerobic benefit to running and biking, when frequency, duration, and intensity are held constant.

Burns Calories. Walking burns approximately 200–300 calories per hour at a brisk pace of 3–4 miles per hour. Walkers burn almost the same number of calories as runners per distance traveled. Walking a mile uses as many calories as running a mile. The difference, of course, is that walking takes a lot longer.

Helps Rehabilitate Injuries. Walking is one of the best exercises for the injured runner. Because your foot never rises far off the ground, you don't strike the pavement hard, and jarring and joint stress are minimized. When you walk you land on your foot with the equivalent of one gravity force; when you run, you land with three to four.

You can walk during your convalescence with almost any running injury. And alternating between running and walking will help you move safely back into full-time running.

Aids Recovery from Hard Work. Dick Beardsley, a close runner-up to Alberto Salazar in the exciting 1982 Boston Marathon, walks between his runs twice a day. Every night before he goes to bed, he walks for 15 or 20 minutes, sometimes even more than that. He reports that it helps him mentally, and he walks the junk out of his legs. Walking is as much a part of his training as going out and pounding the miles.

Serves as a Warm-up for Running. A brisk walk, especially on cold days or in the early morning when you are stiff, warms the muscles, stretches you out, and thus helps minimize injury.

Supplements Running Training. If you walk fast enough or long enough, walking can be used to supplement your running and minimize injury.

DISADVANTAGES OF WALKING

There is really only one major disadvantage of walking for runners: It takes a long time. You have to walk at least twice as long to get the same benefit as running unless you can walk so briskly that you are in your training heart rate range.

HOW FAST, HOW FAR, HOW LONG: WALKING VERSUS RUNNING

Speed. You can walk as fast as you like. How vigorously you walk will depend on your injury, your conditioning, the terrain and weather, and what you want to achieve. Generally, however, a brisk walk of 4 miles per hour (15 minutes per mile) will get your heart rate up into your training range. Some runners will find that on hills they can walk faster than the average jogger runs. But if your conditioning is at the high competitive level, walking won't generate much exercise for you unless you walk up hills or stairs, carry a backpack over rugged terrain, or swing your arms vigorously and really step out. Some older or less fit runner-walkers may be able to reach their training heart rate range at a moderate pace of 3 miles per hour (20 minutes per mile).

Distance. A vigorous walk of 2½ miles is the aerobic equivalent of running 1 mile.

Time. Most people have to walk two to three times as long to get the same benefits from walking as from running. If you can keep your heart rate in your training range for 30 minutes of brisk walking, it is equal to 30 minutes of running in terms of cardiovascular conditioning. The rule of thumb is this: If you can't get your heart rate up for a sustained period of time, you will have to walk for 2 hours or more for it to be the training equivalent of 1 hour of running.

GUIDELINES FOR WALKERS

• Make sure you have well-cushioned, comfortable walking shoes, running shoes, or hiking boots.

• Never walk on your toes. As in running, this can strain your lower legs, ankles, and calves.

• Start with a comfortable speed (about 20 minutes per mile), and try to work up to a fast speed (about 15 minutes per mile). Lengthen your stride and quicken your pace (steps per minute) as you become more accustomed to fast walking. As you go faster, swing your arms vigorously to help increase your heart rate.

• According to Dr. Fred Stutman, author of *The Doctor's Walking Book*, the most comfortable walking position starts with your weight over your feet. Your body should be relaxed and in a slight forward lean, with your knees slightly bent. To utilize your leg muscles properly, use the "heel-toe method." Point your feet straight ahead, bring the leading leg forward in front of your body, and touch the heel of this foot to the ground just before pushing off the ball of your other foot. As you walk, shift your weight forward and bend your knee so that your heel is raised and your toes are in position to push off for the next step.

Keep your posture erect, with your shoulders loose and your hands and forearms carried low. If you hold your arms too high, you'll experience tension in your neck and shoulder muscles. Walk smoothly, putting energy into each step. You'll soon develop a rhythm and stride that's most natural for you.

FOR MORE INFORMATION

Books

The Complete Book of Walking by Charles Kuntzleman (New York: Simon & Schuster, 1979).

The Doctor's Walking Book by Fred A. Stutman, M.D. (New York: Ballantine Books, 1980).

The New Complete Walker by Colin Fletcher (New York: Alfred A. Knopf, 1977).

11 RACE WALKING

The Olympic sport of race walking is a combination of running and walking. The race walker drives with the hips and pumps with the arms to propel the body forward, but a part of one foot is always on the ground. Race walking can be an enjoyable alternative exercise and can also benefit your training. You don't have to race to race walk, in fact most people utilize it as a fitness activity. However, the injured runner who misses competition can enjoy race walking competition. Some runners become converts and never return to the road racing scene; others alternate between the two types of competition.

Here are some of the benefits of race walking:

Increases Aerobic Endurance. Because the race walker is driving the arms powerfully and taking more and longer steps per minute than in walking, race walking really drives the heart rate up and is—if properly done—of equivalent aerobic benefit to running. Thus, 30 minutes of race walking is equal to a 30-minute run.

Burns Calories. A 1979 study by Dr. Robert Gutin, head of the Department of Applied Physiology at Columbia University, demonstrated that race walkers burn more calories than runners at a similar speed because the race walker's upper *and* lower body are working and burning fuel. Running at 7½ minutes per mile and race walking at 10 minutes per mile are about equivalent in effort and burn approximately the same number of calories per hour.

Balances Muscle Development. Race walking strengthens muscles in both the front and back of the legs, while running strengthens only those in the back. Race walking also strengthens other areas not much affected by running: abdominals, buttocks, upper body, arms. Stronger abdominal muscles will help the runner maintain good running posture, and stronger arms and upper body will improve the runner's arm drive. Because race walkers learn to drive their arms really powerfully, the runner who race walks can also improve his or her form and gain an awareness of the value of arm action in increasing running speed. Race walking can also improve a runner's muscular endurance.

Improves Flexibility. As the race walker steps forward with the leg, the hip is pushed forward. This action increases hip flexibility and minimizes hip and back injury for runners.

Helps Rehabilitate Injuries. Probably 90 percent of race walkers are former runners who took up the sport while they were injured and looking for an alternative exercise. In race walking, they found an activity that causes few injuries. Race walking eliminates the jarring action of running, and, because it strengthens both the front and back of the legs, it also minimizes injury caused by muscle imbalances. George Sheehan, M.D., states in *Dr. Sheehan on Running* that "racewalking is the perfect sport for recuperants from some other sports. . . . The ailing athlete who turns to racewalking will soon find himself on the mend."

Supplements Running Training. Race walking can be used to prevent injury and to improve your running. According to Howard Jacobson, author of *Racewalk to Fitness: The Sensible Alternative to Jogging and Running*, "Racewalking, when paired with running, is a form of cross-training which strengthens the adjunct group of muscles, while contributing to aerobic fitness. With the cross-training effect of a combined running and racewalking program you can (1) increase your overall athletic strength, (2) further refine your running style, and (3) better protect yourself from injury. Those runners whom I have put on a cross-training schedule report dramatically improved running times."

DISADVANTAGES OF RACE WALKING

• Wiggling your fanny as you walk down the street looks funny, but perhaps it doesn't look any stranger than running looked before it became accepted in the 1970s. If you can ignore the comments from onlookers, race walking is great exercise.

• There are few race walking coaches, and it is necessary to learn the proper form. In fact, race walkers can be disqualified from races for form faults.

HOW FAST, HOW FAR, HOW LONG: RACE WALKING VERSUS RUNNING

Speed. You race walk faster than you walk, but slower than you run. Some race walkers can race faster than good runners; a top race walker can walk sub-6-minute miles and sub-3-hour marathons. For the average person, race walking pace ranges between 10 and 20 minutes per mile. A brisk race walking pace is about 10 minutes per mile, compared with a fast running pace of approximately 7½ minutes per mile and a walking pace of 15 minutes per mile. As with other aerobic alternatives, you need to walk fast enough to bring your heart rate into your training range.

Distance. You won't have to do as much mileage with race walking as with running to get equal aerobic value because you'll be working just as hard, but at a slower speed. Depending on your relative skills as a runner and race walker, you'll cover approximately 25 percent less distance per hour race walking than running. Three miles of race walking will be approximately equal to 4 miles of running.

Time. If you use proper technique, you can replace running aerobically minute for minute with race walking.

GUIDELINES FOR RACE WALKERS

• Warm up properly before starting your workout. Don't just stretch your legs, but exercise to loosen up your shoulders, arms, and hips.

• Wear well-cushioned running shoes for race walking.

• Proper technique is important. Dr. Barry Block noted in *Running & Fitness* that it "allows the racewalker to utilize the entire body to maximum advantage. The hips, for instance, should be extended to their maximum with each stride to increase the distance covered. This downward and forward extension gives the racewalker a characteristic 'swivel-hipped' gait. The knee serves as a forward driving force, starting from a backward position at toe-off until becoming fully extended at heel contact. Arms should remain bent to the perpendicular (90 degrees), shortening the pendulum-like swing and allowing a quicker pace. Arms and shoulders act in the opposite rhythm of your hips, helping balance the body. Fists should be loosely clenched and cross your body at mid-chest with your elbows barely touching your ribs."

Technically, race walking differs from running and walking in that one foot must always be in contact with the ground and the knee must be straight when pushing off. If a highly conditioned runner who suddenly takes up race walking isn't careful, the straightening of the knee at a fast pace can cause hyperextension and injury to the knee.

FOR MORE INFORMATION

Books

Racewalk to Fitness: The Sensible Alternative to Jogging and Running by Howard Jacobson (New York: Simon & Schuster, 1980).

Organization

Walkers Club of America
445 East Eighty-sixth Street
New York, NY 10028

12 CROSS-COUNTRY SKIING

Cross-country skiing is an exciting aerobic sport. You can ski on well-prepared tracks or head off through the woods to tour through unbroken snow. In New England and other places where there is snow in the winter, you will find many runners who both run and ski. Dr. Joan Ullyot explained in her book, *Running Free,* that "cross-country skiing is by far the best substitute for running, demanding the same qualities of endurance, cardiovascular conditioning, and leg strength that runners need. In addition, skiing demands a certain grace and balance that are optional in running, as well as considerable upper body strength, which most runners lack. Thus, while cross-country skiing is easy to learn and fun to do, as well as inexpensive, it ends up being even more demanding than running. In fact, cross-country skiers regard running as a second-best alternative to their own sport, something they practice only in the summer, to keep in shape."

Art Stegen, who coaches both cross-country running and cross-country skiing at New Paltz (NY) High School, compared the two sports in an article in *New York Running News:* "The psychological and physiological demands of distance running and nordic skiing are obviously alike. In fact, oxygen uptake tests have shown that nordic skiers achieve slightly higher values at peak levels than runners. This is partly due to the extra effort required from skiers' arms. In almost all other physical tests, runners and skiers show similar results. Energy costs and fluid needs are nearly equal. Training patterns are alike: interval, distance, and fartlek work are common to both, as are bounding drills and strength building exercises. The degrees of aerobic and anaerobic conditioning demanded by the two disciplines are comparable, as well." According to Stegen, there are two basic differences between running and cross-country skiing: The technique for proper skiing must be mastered, and much less shock and stress is placed on the muscles in skiing.

Here are some of the benefits of cross-country skiing:

Increases Aerobic Endurance. Several studies have shown that top cross-country skiers score higher than top runners in tests measuring maximal oxygen uptake. In his latest in a series of aerobics books, *The Aerobics Program for Well-Being*, Dr. Kenneth Cooper ranks cross-country skiing as the number 1 aerobic activity, because, as he explains, "you have more muscles involved than just the legs, and any time you get more muscles involved, you get more aerobic benefit. But there are other advantages that cross-country skiing has over most other aerobic sports. The fact that this activity is usually done at relatively high altitudes and in cold weather adds additional strain on the body, and that means a more rigorous workout. Finally, it's necessary to wear heavier clothing in cross-country skiing than in most other aerobic activities, and so you have an overload principle at work—an added weight on the body which further enhances the aerobic effect."

Burns Calories. Skiers who travel at faster speeds than runners or over more rugged terrain will burn as many or more calories per hour of effort as runners.

Balances Muscle Development. While cross-country skiing, the injured runner strengthens all major muscle groups used in running. In addition, he or she strengthens muscle groups that will help to minimize injury: upper body, arms, abdominals, buttocks, and quadriceps.

Improves Flexibility. The gliding action of skiing helps stretch out the muscles in the back and back of the legs, which are tightened with running.

Helps Rehabilitate Injuries. According to Dr. Joan Ullyot, "Almost all running injuries respond well to skiing, because the gliding movement eliminates jarring while exercising muscles and joints." Because it involves very little pounding on the knees, joints, and muscles, top cross-country competitors can stay at the top of their sport well into their forties, much longer than competitive runners.

Offers a Break from Bad Weather. Snow and ice bring two obstacles to the runner, slippery footing and running paths narrowed by snow. To avoid injuries caused by slippery footing, and to avoid the hassle of sharing roads full of snow with car traffic and getting splashed by salty slush, you can head for the woods on cross-country skis. Take advantage of a large snowfall rather than let it ruin your training routine.

Provides a Change of Pace. Cross-country skiing allows you to take a mental break from the strict discipline of running and explore the beautiful scenery of wooded lands filled with freshly fallen snow. As Bob Woodward observed in *Running & Fitness*, "Once you get into advanced technique, you begin to understand what makes cross-country skiing so addictive. There's a flowing feeling as you glide over the snow. There's an exhilarating feeling of total exhaustion after a good workout, and a sense of satisfaction as your whole body firms up. There're the mentally-toughening uphills and spirit-lifting downhills. Cross-country skiing is demanding in a very different sense from running. On a long-distance run, your body is tested by pounding; on a long ski, your mind is tested over and over again."

Encourages Family Participation. As Europeans have known for decades, cross-country skiing is a great family sport. According to Woodward, there has been a great deal of talk about running as a family sport, but surveys show that the majority of runners are adults. Cross-country skiing, on the other hand, has something for everyone. Kids who are easily bored can find plenty of steep downhills, jumps, snowball fights, and mischief to keep them happily involved in cross-country. Unlike running, which is criticized as a potentially dangerous activity for a child's growing musculoskeletal system because of the pounding it involves, cross-country skiing is a safe activity for young people.

Enhances Running Form. The arm action used in skiing helps the runner understand the value of the arm thrust in running. It also improves the upper-body and arm muscles needed to execute powerful arm drives while running at fast speeds.

Supplements Running Training. Combined with a weight training program, cross-country skiing may return you to the roads in the spring in better shape than you left them in autumn. Adds Art Stegen, "As a high school coach without an indoor track program, I convince most of my distance runners to ski during the winter. Those who ski often maintain a higher level of fitness over the winter than those who try to continue running. My runners are able to compete successfully well into the summer months, at a time when those from other teams are over-raced or overtrained."

DISADVANTAGES OF CROSS-COUNTRY SKIING

• You need equipment—poles, shoes, skis—and lessons for the first few outings. But the cost of renting equipment is relatively low, and the technique is surprisingly easy to learn. Until you master reasonably good technique, however, you may have difficulty reaching your training heart rate range.

• It is difficult to get a sustained workout in deep, unpacked snow.

HOW FAST, HOW FAR, HOW LONG: CROSS-COUNTRY SKIING VERSUS RUNNING

Speed. A top cross-country skier traversing fast tracks can travel a 10-kilometer distance faster than a runner. But an unskilled skier covering rugged terrain will travel much slower than a runner. Speed depends on many factors: skill, equipment, terrain, surface. The important thing is not how fast you go, but rather that you exercise within your training heart rate range.

Distance. You may ski more or less distance in an hour than you would run, depending on the same factors that govern your speed. Popular local races are 10–40 kilometers. Most serious Olympic-level competition is 5–20 kilometers for women, 15–50 kilometers for men. Races over 50 kilometers, which are quite popular among average racers, are considered marathons.

Time. Because of the variety of terrain involved and the many factors affecting speed, what is important in cross-country skiing is how much time you exercise. Count minutes, not mileage. If you are able to keep your pulse in your training range, the time involved in equivalent training is the same as running, thus you can replace running aerobically minute for minute with cross-country skiing.

GUIDELINES FOR CROSS-COUNTRY SKIERS

• Warm up thoroughly before skiing. Stretch the same muscles you use for running, and, as with race walking, stretch muscles in the upper body, arms, and hips as well.

• Good equipment and good technique are important. According to Bob Woodward, "Any beginning cross-country skier should consider lessons first and foremost. Running on skis doesn't do the job. Cross-country technique is more like ice-skating technique, a fluid, graceful motion that drives down the ski track. The strides are longer than running strides, with a more dramatic shift in weight from one foot to the other." Skiers glide along a trail, lifting each foot high while pulling along with ski poles. To go uphill, cross-country skiers actually sprint, using the poles to pull them along while taking small jogging steps. Some skiers also run downhill, but most cross-country courses have only small, rolling, uphill and downhill paths.

• Competitive runners switching to cross-country skiing would be wise to keep on running occasionally throughout the winter, unless they are forced to stop because of an injury. Runs every two or three days will supplement the skiing. Cut back your mileage in proportion to the time added with the new activity, but don't lose your running legs.

• Ease into cross-country skiing, even if you are a veteran skier returning for another winter of enjoyable aerobic exercise. Remember that your cardiovascular system will be able to handle much more stress than your musculoskeletal system. If you ski too much too soon, you could find yourself very sore the next day.

GUIDELINES FOR COMPETITIVE TRAINING

Cross-country skiers use running, with intervals and hill work, to train for their sport. Most high-school and college teams start workouts in the late fall, when the roads and ski trails are free of snow. Workouts consist of long-distance runs of up to 12 miles, interspersed with interval training. Runners who are forced to lay off because of injury can use the same training program they would have followed if they were running. However, they should count minutes instead of mileage.

Sally O'Connell's experience is a good example of how a competitive runner can use cross-country skiing as an alternative training exercise. She moved to Boston in the winter of 1982, just in time for a blizzard that buried all her newly found running trails.

She learned to cross-country ski, and even after her running paths were plowed, she continued her new sport as a way of taking a break and protecting herself from the frequent shock-related injuries she got most winters after a hard summer and fall of road racing. Eventually, Sally learned the skills well enough to use this alternative exercise two or three times a week as part of her foundation training for the Boston Marathon. Once a week she would ski for 30–60 minutes over a fast, flat course—a tempo workout in track language. On weekends she would ski for 1 hour of mild fartlek, including bounding hard up hills for power workouts. Other days she would ski for long training sessions of 2–3 hours. She followed this program for the months of December and January and cut her running mileage from 60–70 miles per week to 30–40. The change in routine gave her a physical and mental break. In February she gradually increased her running mileage and decreased her cross-country ski time until she was back up to running 70 miles a week. When she returned to the track for sharpening sessions, Sally was shocked to find that her times were as fast as when she had left in the fall. The cross-country skiing provided her with solid aerobic and anaerobic training, and also increased her upper-body strength, which helped her to run faster.

FOR MORE INFORMATION

Books

The New Cross-Country Ski Book by John Caldwell (New York: Bantam Books, 1976).

Cross-Country Skiing Guide by the publishers of *Nordic World* (Mountain View, CA: World Publishing, 1978).

Magazine

Cross-Country Skier
Box 1203
Brattleboro, VT 05301

Part V
MANAGEMENT OF INJURY

13 TREATMENT OPTIONS

When you are injured, you can respond in one of four ways: ignore it and run through it, often making it worse; quit running and pray that it will go away; attempt self-treatment; or seek medical help. Most runners deal with an injury in that order: ignoring it, quitting for a few days, attempting self-treatment, and, finally, seeing a doctor.

Guidelines for running through injuries and coming back after a layoff are detailed in Chapters 4 and 5. Methods for self-treatment are discussed in the following chapters. Here, we will examine four key questions that injured runners ask: When do I need to see a doctor? Which type of sports-medicine specialist should I consult? How do I choose a doctor? What should I expect from him or her?

WHEN TO SEE A DOCTOR

According to Dr. Gabe Mirkin and Marshall Hoffman in *The Sportsmedicine Book*, you should consult a sports-medicine specialist for

"1. All traumatic joint injuries. All injuries to a joint and its ligaments should be examined by a sportsmedicine physician because these injuries have the potential of becoming permanent and debilitating if proper treatment is not administered.

2. Any injury accompanied by severe pain. Pain is nature's way of talking to you and when it speaks loudly, you had better listen.

3. Any pain in a joint or bone that persists for more than two weeks. These tissues are the ones in which the most serious injuries occur.

4. Any injury that doesn't heal in three weeks. All injuries that don't heal should be checked for a structural abnormality that may have caused them. Sometimes an injury may not heal because you won't rest it.

5. Any injury that you feel should be checked. If you are concerned about an injury, you should always ask for help.

6. Any infection in or under the skin manifested by pus, red streaks, swollen lymph nodes, or fever. Untreated infections may lead to serious complications, and since antibiotics generally bring relief quickly, it is foolish not to receive treatment."

Further guidelines:

- Dr. Weisenfeld's rule: If the pain is with you from the first step, the problem is usually not biomechanical. If it comes on into the run, after the run, or the next day, it's probably a biomechanical problem, and a sports-medicine specialist should be consulted.

- If pain doesn't diminish with a short (three- or four-day) layoff, or if it worsens during a layoff, see a doctor.

- If an inflamed tendon (tendinitis) does not respond to rest or ice in ten days, see a doctor.

WHAT TYPE OF SPORTS-MEDICINE SPECIALIST TO CONSULT

As we have mentioned, virtually every runner is injured and thus must seek some sort of treatment. Many end up having to make a sometimes confusing choice: Whom do I go to? According to a study by California podiatrist Joe Ellis of nearly 11,000 runners who had experienced running injuries, some 52 percent went to a doctor. The most common type of doctor visited was a podiatrist, followed by a family physician, and an orthopedist.

If you have an injury, you have two options in terms of medical treatment: Seek help from your family doctor or internist, or consult a "sports-medicine specialist," a new breed of doctors and other trained personnel who specialize to some degree in treating athletes. Until the fitness boom of the 1970s, few doctors exercised, and most of their patients were sedentary. The running and fitness revolution brought with it a demand for more than the traditional doctor's remedy: Take aspirin and stop running. Runners want to keep running and will seek specialists to help them cope with their injuries so they can.

According to Robert Kropf, "one must recognize the uniqueness of the sports-medicine field in relation to other areas of medical specialty. The most startling difference is that sports medicine emerged to its present state of prominence due to a change of lifestyle. People all over the world began improving the quality of their lives by exercising. This is in stark contrast to other branches of medicine, which originated in response to a new disease, new treatment, or new diagnostic methods for present medical conditions. The second major difference is the type of patient one sees in a sports-medicine clinic—they are usually healthy!

"Sports medicine is a total system of health care for the athlete and for those who wish to improve their health by exercising. This system includes sports specialists in many diversified professions who work together to provide complete care for the physically active. Some of these services are as follows:

- Consultations for those who wish to begin exercising safely.
- Prescreening examinations to find areas of weakness where an injury may occur.

- Early diagnosis of athletic injuries.
- Prompt treatment of injury.
- Total rehabilitation to insure the safest and quickest return to athletic activity from an injury.

"Inherent in all the above services is the communication between the specialist and the patient. This provides a basis for educating the patient on why the injury happened, how to treat it, when to return to athletic activity, and how to prevent the injury from reoccurring."

Who is a sports-medicine specialist? There is a problem with this term, and that is that anyone—including some quacks—can claim to be one. Allan J. Ryan, M.D., editor-in-chief of *The Physician and Sportsmedicine*, observes, "There are very few medical schools or residencies which offer training in sportsmedicine. Without courses, there is no way that you could give an examination to certify special competence in the field. Thus, sportsmedicine is not a recognized specialty such as internal medicine or pediatrics." The athlete may benefit from medical personnel from a wide range of specialties: The family practitioner, internist, orthopedist, neurosurgeon, podiatrist, gynecologist are just a few. Most MDs who become very good sports doctors do so because of their special interest in sports, engagement in continuing education programs, and personal experience. These physicians must be aware of the current state of knowledge in their specialty and its application to the athlete. They must know their treatment limitations and work with other specialists in an effort to provide the best possible service to the athlete. The practice of sports medicine is by no means limited to treatment by a physician. A large number of specialists are involved in this field, including physical therapists, exercise physiologists, sports psychologists, scientists, computer specialists, and biomechanics and engineering specialists, to name a few.

The following characteristics should be requirements for a sports-medicine specialist for runners:

- He or she should be a runner, or at the very least a runner at heart.
- He or she should have experience treating many athletes, especially runners.
- He or she should have a good background—through formal schooling and personal research—in general medicine and exercise. Although there is no separate field of sports medicine today, each medical specialty offers extensive courses on athletic injuries as related to it. The sports-medicine specialist you consult should have that continuing education background.
- He or she should be recommended by others: experienced runners, running organizations, your family doctor, another respected sports-medicine specialist. You can get lists of doctors who are interested in sports medicine from the American College of Sports Medicine, the American Academy of Podiatric Sports Medicine, the American Orthopaedic Society for Sports Medicine, and the orthopedic and sports section of the Physical Therapy Association. Local running clubs and podiatric and medical societies may also have lists of doctors in the field.

HOW TO CHOOSE A SPECIALIST

Choosing the right specialist for your injury is often a problem. Whatever your injury, you are likely to get a different opinion from different specialists. A podiatrist is likely to say your hip hurts because of a problem in your foot structure; a chiropractor that you need your spine realigned; a physical therapist that you need special exercises to correct relative weaknesses; an orthopedist that you have a structural problem; a shoe salesperson that you need different shoes, and so on.

Your family physician or a sports-oriented internist can screen and refer you to the appropriate type of specialist for your problem. You can also go to a private sports-medicine clinic or one associated with a hospital, where a team of specialists pool their talents to help injured athletes. Ideally, you will be referred to a competent sports-medicine specialist who will consult with other specialists if necessary. Beware of anyone who refuses to listen to what other disciplines have to offer. In the past few doctors were willing to "share" their patients (and fees) with others. Now, more cooperation is evident as runners demand more and more specialized treatment. James C. G. Coniff noted in his article "Who Do You Turn To?" in *The Runner:* "A growing spirit of teamwork on behalf of runners in trouble has begun to overshadow the ancient antagonisms among medical specialists." Dr. Weisenfeld, for example, works in cooperation with several specialists, including orthopedists, osteopaths, physical therapists, acupuncturists, chiropractors, endocrinologists, internists, physical rehabilitation specialists, and other podiatrists.

WHAT TO EXPECT FROM A SPORTS-MEDICINE SPECIALIST

You should expect two things from a sports-medicine specialist:

Diagnosis. The specialist should carefully examine your history and consider all the possible causes of your injury. An X ray may be taken if you suspect a stress fracture. (*Note:* Don't forget that *you,* not the doctor, own the X ray; don't be afraid to ask for it. The X ray is your personal property; it can be obtained from your doctor with a written release from you.) The next step is a "hands-on" examination, which may include tests for leg-length discrepancy, biomechanical imbalances, and so on. The doctor should conclude with a complete explanation—in words that you can understand—of the treatment he or she recommends. Don't let the doctor hurry you out to get to the next patient. Ask questions if you don't understand the explanation. Keep this point in mind—your first visit is for diagnosis, not treatment. You may decide to think over the treatment options before starting them.

Treatment. After considering the treatment options the doctor offers, you may be wise to discuss them with your coach. Be conservative. Don't accept drugs, especially injections, until other options, for example, physical therapy, have been tried. Never accept surgery as a solution without a second or third opinion. The doctor should give you directions for treatment using the options discussed in the following chapters. He or she should also give you some guidelines on how to alter your training during treatment.

Whoever you decide to use as your sports-medicine specialist, give his or her treatment a chance. Few treatment choices result in immediate recovery. If orthotics are prescribed along with special exercises, give them a good try. Many runners are impatient and don't follow a prescribed treatment properly; they then complain that it didn't work and search for another specialist. Remember, too, that every doctor can't cure every patient. Dr. Weisenfeld is happy if 80 percent of his patients are cured with his treatment. If a doctor can't cure your ailment, he or she should refer you to another sports-medicine specialist who may be able to help you by looking at your problem from a different perspective.

SPORTS-MEDICINE SPECIALISTS

Here is a summary of what some of the leading disciplines in sports medicine (listed alphabetically) have to offer the runner.

Acupuncturist

The Chinese method of acupuncture involves using needles to pierce peripheral nerves in order to ease pain and heal injuries. Check credentials: Only specially trained and licensed physicians can call themselves acupuncturists.

Chiropractor (D.C.)

Believing that misalignment of the vertebrae is responsible for most disease processes, chiropractors specialize in manipulation as treatment for abnormal nerve function and muscle spasm. The chiropractor applies pressure with his or her hands to move misaligned joints in the proper direction. A chiropractor is not licensed to prescribe medicine, inject drugs, or do any type of surgery. Competent chiropractors will refer patients to orthopedists if they suspect structural damage and to podiatrists if they suspect that weaknesses in the foot are causing misalignment. Chiropractor Seymour "Mac" Goldstein, who is the attending medical specialist for the Colgate Women's Games, believes that if he can't help you in three visits for "adjustments," you should look elsewhere for help. Beware of chiropractors who want you to visit them several times a week for a lengthy period of time. Chiropractors have been particularly helpful to runners with back, groin, hip, and hamstring problems.

Orthopedist (M.D.)

The orthopedic surgeon is a medical doctor who specializes in musculoskeletal disorders of the joints and bones. Such a specialist should always be consulted when a fracture or structural damage is suspected. A competent orthopedist will help you avoid surgery by suggesting rehabilitation exercises and referring you to a physical therapist (for muscle and joint rehabilitation), podiatrist (if foot problems are suspected as the cause of knee, back, and hip pain), or other specialist.

Osteopath (D.O.)

Osteopaths are medical doctors trained to use manipulation to treat injuries. They have been particularly helpful to runners with hip and back pain.

Physiatrist (M.D.)

The physiatrist is a specialist in rehabilitation medicine. This specialist uses treatments designed to relieve pain sufficiently to utilize exercise as a rehabilitation technique. Physiatrists utilize whirlpool treatments and ultrasound, and work in conjunction with physical therapists.

Physical Therapist (R.P.T.)

Physical therapists are allied health professionals who are licensed within their respective states after attending special colleges accredited by the American Physical Therapy Association.

According to Robert Kropf, "physical therapy is the evaluation and treatment of musculoskeletal dysfunction (pain, loss of movement, decreased muscle strength). Physical therapists use many types of modalities—heat, cold, ultrasound, diathermy, electricity, massage, and specifically designed exercises. The mere application of one or more of these modalities does not constitute a physical therapy treatment. Physical therapists are allied health professionals who have the expertise to coordinate modalities into a total treatment and rehabilitation plan. They view the patient as a whole, realizing that an injury is, more often than not, the weak link in the biomechanical chain of the area which has broken down due to other factors. A complete plan of rehabilitation is designed, which provides direct treatment to the site of the injury and takes into account any other contributing factors, to insure the quickest and safest return to activity.

"In most states, physical therapists provide a vital link in the sports-medicine field, for they work upon referral of a patient from an orthopedist, osteopath, internist, and podiatrist. However, there are six states presently where therapists do not require referrals for treatment, and in many states they are able to see patients independently for evaluation."

Podiatrist (D.P.M.)

A podiatrist is a medically trained specialist in foot function and injuries. Pioneer podiatrists such as Dr. Richard Schuster helped popularize their specialty as a treatment option for injured runners long before the term *sports medicine* was coined. Podiatrists are most effective in the treatment of injuries from the knee down that are caused by biomechanically weak feet or unequal leg length. If runners didn't pound the ground with three times the force of their body weight, 1,000 times per mile, podiatrists wouldn't have become leaders in the treatment of runners' injuries. The podiatrist uses a variety of treatments, including taping, ultrasound, whirlpool, and exercise, but may also prescribe orthotics (see Chaper 14). Competent podiatrists will refer patients to orthopedists if structural damage is suspected and to physical therapists if a structured program of injury rehabilitation is needed.

TREATMENT OPTIONS

Whether the injured runner visits a sports-medicine specialist or attempts self-treatment, he or she can choose from many treatment options. The runner's first task is dealing with the immediate problem of inflammation, which is present with most injuries. As Dr. Joan Ullyot describes in *Women's Running*, "the immediate response of the body to the damage is the same: a local outpouring of fluids and cells release substances that cause an inflammatory response, with more leakage of blood cells and lymph—and the results are the classic five signals: heat, redness, pain, swelling and loss of function."

As most runners already know, disability can be minimized by keeping the swelling down through RICE (rest, ice, compression, elevation) if done immediately after the injury occurs and continued for a day or two. Rest means staying off the injury for a while; ice, or cold treatment, is explained in the next section; compression involves wrapping the injured area; and elevation means raising the injured area above the heart level. After 48 hours you should start promoting circulation, because increased blood flow to the injured area will help remove waste products and fluid, which speeds healing. Heat, massage, gentle exercise, and ultrasound will hasten this process, though some think that only ice treatment should be used.

The various treatments that can be used by your doctor, physical therapist, or in some cases yourself, do one or more of three things: heal the injury, rehabilitate the runner, treat the cause of the injury. Here we will examine some of the most often prescribed treatment options for runners.

Cold Treatments

Cold treatment (cryotherapy) is the most common treatment for injured runners. It lessens pain, reduces inflammation, decreases blood flow, and brings down swelling and fluid build-up in the injured area. It is often used in combination with aspirin, which also reduces pain and inflammation. Cold treatment temporarily relieves muscle spasms because it numbs and calms the irritated nerve fibers around the affected muscles. Ice is most often used in cryotherapy. It is applied immediately after an injury to minimize inflammation and frequently thereafter for at least 24 hours and throughout injury rehabilitation. Cold treatment is advised for inflammation experienced by the athlete running through a minor injury or coming back from an injury. Although heat treatment is most often used 48 hours after an injury, the use of cold is still advised directly following the run.

Cold treatment can be used passively or in combination with gentle movement to aid healing. According to Ben Benjamin, Ph.D., author of *Listen to Your Pain*, "ice can be very effective as treatment, especially when applied immediately after an injury. Ice permits your body to heal quickly in two ways: it promotes even greater blood circulation than heat, and it numbs the pain so that you can move the injured area. The latter is beneficial because the best healing takes place when you actively move your injured part. Movement allows the new-forming tissue to remain pliable and healthy. . . . Chill the injured area for about six to twelve minutes, until it gets numb. Then begin to move it, starting with small movements and gradually increasing your range of motion. Remember to move *gently,* and without putting weight on the injury. When the numbness wears off and you start feeling the pain again, apply the ice and repeat the whole procedure. It is the movement part of the ice therapy that makes it so effective. Moving stimulates proper healing by increasing blood circulation and preventing abnormal scar tissue from forming."

Some caution must be exercised when using cold therapy:
- Cold masks pain, which protects you from further injury. Never run or do any strenuous exercise while you are numb from cryotherapy.
- Be wary of frostbite. Don't leave ice on the bare skin for too long at a time or it will burn you or cause frostbite. Be sure that something is always placed between your skin and the cold application, and be alert to signs of frostbite.
- Cold therapy is not recommended if you are allergic to cold or have diabetes, circulatory problems, rheumatic disease, or Raynaud's disease.

There are several methods of applying cold:

Ice Packs. Ice packs are best for immediate treatment of injuries involving severe pain and swelling. Apply a pack for 15–20 minutes with compression and elevation. Then use for 15–20 minutes on and 15–20 minutes off for the first 3–4 hours after an injury. Finally, apply the pack for 20 minutes, three times a day for 7 days.

You can use various types of ice packs:
- Place crushed ice between two towels.

- Fill an ice bag with ice.
- Buy reusable commercial ice packs that are frozen in your freezer, or chemical bags that mix to produce cold.
- Freeze a wet terry cloth hand towel, fold in a square, and wrap in plastic.

Ice Towels. An ice towel is good for large areas, such as the lower back and hamstrings. Soak a towel in 40° F ice water and place it on the injured area. As it warms up, resoak it. Continue the process for 15–20 minutes.

Ice Massages. The best method to apply cold to an injured area is ice massage. Physical therapist Ted Corbitt, a 1952 U.S. Olympic marathoner, recommends this technique: Freeze ice in a cup for easy application; put Vaseline or baby oil over the injured area to minimize burning; use a rubber glove for comfort while applying; and gently massage the area on and around the injury for 10–15 minutes. Be very careful not to allow the ice to touch bare skin for too long at one time. It is important to keep the ice moving to provide a massaging effect. This treatment is most often used 48 hours after severe injuries and for minor pains.

Cold Water. Cold water, especially cold running water, can help minimize pain and swelling. Cold baths or whirlpools can be especially helpful for sciatica. Run cold water over the injured area with a shower nozzle or garden hose. Once you recover from the shock, your body will adjust to it and will feel good. This method will help you run through injuries, prevent injuries, and recover from tough races and workouts. Jack Foster, an Olympic marathoner in his forties, splashes his legs with a garden hose after any long or fast run to minimize injury.

Heat Treatments

Heat treatment (thermotherapy) increases blood circulation, thus speeding the healing process, by causing the blood vessels to open wider. Thermotherapy is *not* the preferred initial first-aid treatment—cold is. It is used approximately 48 hours after injury, following cold treatment, but only if swelling has lessened. The use of heat too soon after an injury, or right after a run if the exercise causes inflammation, will delay recovery. Heat is helpful to relieve muscle spasms and sore muscles.

There are several methods for applying heat:

Hot Baths and Whirlpools. Hot baths and whirlpools are among the best ways to maintain and increase health and recover from injuries, though ice is best for their initial treatment. Water has fifty times greater heat conductivity than air, and water baths bring heat into the body or conduct it away much faster than air at the same temperature.

Hot tubs promote recovery, and their effect is greater the longer and more deeply immersed you are in them. Hot baths gradually increase the work of your heart, circulatory system, and metabolism. Fifteen minutes in a hot tub, especially one with whirlpool sprays, will greatly aid your circulatory system, help carry away fluids in damaged tissue, and relax muscles. A sauna or hot shower exposes your body to too much air to match the benefits of the hot tub. The whirlpool temperature should be set at 90–100° F. If your heart is immersed, lower the temperature and be alert for signs of dizziness. A whirlpool bath is especially helpful to a runner coming back after a long layoff because it relieves muscle stiffness. The result is maximum massage to the Achilles tendons, ligaments, points of muscle strain, and other foot or ankle injuries.

Hydrocollater Packs. Hydrocollater packs are available in drugstores. They are filled with a dry silica gel, which expands and absorbs heat when placed in hot water. They are covered with cloth or several layers of towels to protect the skin from burning and are used for about 10–20 minutes per application. At least eight layers of toweling should be placed between the pack and the skin to prevent burns. Care should be taken over desensitized areas of skin or any metal implants. Moist heat is better for muscle relaxation because it has a deeper penetration than dry heat, such as infrared lamps. "Hot" packs should not be used for more than 20–30 minutes at a time.

Hot Water Bottles. Hot water bottles are rubber bags that should be half-filled with hot water and wrapped in a cloth or towels to prevent burning. They are placed on the injured area for 10–20 minutes, as with the hydrocollater.

Hot Towels. Soak a towel in hot water and wrap it around the injured part for 10–20 minutes. As a second option, after wrapping the injured area with a hot towel for 3 or 4 minutes, rub in a heat-producing ointment and wrap again with a hot wet towel. Then, use a heating pad for 15–20 minutes.

Electric Heating Pads. You can wrap an electric heating pad around the injured area for 10–20 minutes.

Heat Lamps. Heat lamps are another form of dry heat: They should be used with care. Do not expose yourself for more than 20 or 30 minutes or use if you have sensitive skin or poor circulation.

Note: Do not use electric heat in conjunction with moist heat because of the potential for electric shock.

Electrotherapy
Electrical Muscle Stimulation. High-voltage electrotherapy uses low amperage and thus safely allows for deep muscle contractions. The use of this machinery is particularly helpful when muscles are tight or in spasm following an injury. The deep muscle relaxation promoted causes an increase in circulation through the muscle and flushes waste products away. This treatment is also frequently used for decreasing swelling, muscle strain, and tendinitis.

Diathermy. Diathermy is a type of deep heating that penetrates into the body's tissues. It is produced through high-frequency electricity, which causes increases in blood flow to the injured area and removal of waste products. It is typically used for lower-back and hamstring strains and bursitis, and helps relieve muscle spasm and cramping.

Ultrasound. Ultrasound is an electrical modality that produces sound waves, causing mild heat to penetrate deep into an injured area. Ultrasound converts high-frequency electrical waves into sound waves that are transmitted through contact with the skin, a lubricant, and a metal transmitter head. Ultrasound is typically used for the treatment of bursitis, muscle strains, ligament strains, neuromas, and to help break up scar adhesions.

Transcutaneous Electrical Nerve Stimulation (TENS). TENS are portable, battery-operated, low-voltage electrical units. Electrical charges are sent from the battery-operated pack to the skin via 2–4 carbon electrodes. Low-voltage electricity is used to stimulate the nervous system, which activates the release of endorphins and enkephalins, the body's natural painkillers. This device is used to treat cases of chronic pain, to minimize pain after surgery, and, recently, to aid in the healing of fractures.

The Laser. The helium-neon cold laser is one single-defined wave length of light finely focused to the area of skin on which it is being directed. This is low-intensity light energy that is absorbed through the skin into the body, where it is converted to heat energy. The laser causes an increase in circulation, a decrease in spasm, and what Russian scientists call a "balance of the biological field." It is believed that each part of our body has an unique biological field that can be disturbed by an injury, and that the low-power laser stimulates the body mechanisms to return the biological field to normal. Treatment is painless and safe, and has been found effective with wound healing (blisters), fracture healing, tendinitis, bursitis, and arthritic conditions. Cold laser has been used in the Soviet Union for over ten years. The only danger associated with its use is the damage to the eyes that could result if one looks directly into the beam of light.

Massage

Massage both prevents and heals injuries. Most top European runners get regular massages, as do competitive cyclists. Massage was considered a key training aid for Finland's Lasse Viren, the four-time Olympic gold-medal winner. The elite Nike-sponsored Athletics West team, including Alberto Salazar and Mary Decker, has a full-time masseur who regularly massages their top runners.

A good massage will last from 15 to 30 minutes. Use a lubricant, and always massage toward the heart. Jock Semple, long-time Boston Marathon official and physical therapist, massages first below and then above the injury, and believes that massage "helps the circulation and gets the blood flowing through the injured area and back to the heart." He recommends massaging your legs while in the tub after long runs. Massage relieves muscle spasm, increases circulation, loosens sore muscles, and relaxes the body. It is used 48 hours after an injury to promote circulation to the injured area. Massage can delay healing if it is used too soon after injury.

Physical therapist Carl Mailhot noted in an interview in *Running & Fitness* that "massage returns the homeostasis or internal stability of soft muscle tissue and normal muscle balance. In addition it improves body flexibility and tone, which results in stronger musculature and increased bodily balance." Perhaps massage's key benefit to runners is the prevention of injury. A good massage helps you recover from a hard workout. Paula Mara Lyons, a registered occupational therapist, believes that "a post-run massage can top off the run and take total advantage of the running experience. Massage relieves the muscles of lactic acid while realigning those muscles used during the run. Massage is a natural completion of the running experience."

Massage is used daily by those fortunate enough to have a full-time masseuse or masseur available. Other athletes have a massage one to three times a week on a regular basis. Massage is most beneficial when used regularly, but the average runner will benefit from periodic massages to help him or her recover from hard training bouts and injury.

Among the many massage techniques are the following:

Deep Massage. Techniques such as Swedish massage are deep in pressure and at times will be uncomfortable, perhaps slightly painful. Vigorous, long strokes are used along with kneading. These techniques are helpful in increasing blood circulation to injured areas and releasing tension built up in the muscles.

Acupressure. Athletes in China have had success with acupressure for years. They believe it relieves pain as well as improves the flexibility and tone of muscles. The finger or knuckle is used to stimulate "pressure points," which are areas in the body where tension collects. "Massaging" these areas breaks up the tension and relieves the pain.

Shiatsu. Shiatsu is a form of massage perfected by the Japanese; it also uses thumb pressure applied to key pressure points to promote healing and relaxation.

Rolfing. The rolfing method uses heavy pressure to realign the body structure. Typically, ten weekly sessions are used to "reshape" the body and relieve tension.

Reflexology. The technique of reflexology is based on the theory that every important organ in the body relates to a certain point in the foot. By massaging that area of the foot, injuries in the corresponding body part can be treated.

Deep Friction Massage. In deep friction massage, pressure is applied at the exact spot of the injury with a constant back-and-forth movement across the painful area. Pressure is maintained for 5–10 minutes and may be painful at first, but the pain diminishes as treatment continues. The purpose of this treatment is to break down scar tissue, which would prevent proper healing. This type of massage should only be attempted by a highly qualified physical therapist.

Myotherapy. Firm, steady pressure is used in myotherapy to break up "trigger points," thus releasing tension and dispersing pain.

All of these treatments should be performed by a well-trained professional, or damage may result. If you are seeking a professional massage to help you recover from injury, you should make sure your massage therapist is certified by the American Massage and Therapy Association or a similar professional organization.

Manipulation

Trained personnel, such as chiropractors, osteopaths, and physical therapists, use manipulation to restore the proper alignment of bones by putting pressure on various joints. Usually manipulation will help you either right away or not at all.

Trigger Point Injections

Trigger points are local tender spots of degenerated muscle tissue in the skeletal muscle. They can produce severe pain or muscle spasm. The pain may radiate down the back and extremities and up the neck and back of the head. Runners are most susceptible to trigger points in the legs and back. Trigger points can be treated with deep friction massage or physical therapy. If that doesn't work, trigger point injection may be utilized by a trained medical specialist. An anesthetic such as lidocaine, procaine, or novocaine is injected into the trigger point to break up the degenerated tissue. This can be very painful, but effective. The treatment is followed on succeeding days by electrical stimulation to relax the muscle. No exercise or prolonged sitting or standing are allowed during treatment. Therapy is followed by a program of relaxation and stretching exercises and a gradual return to a normal running schedule.

Surgery

Surgery should be a last resort, and the need for surgery should always be confirmed by a second opinion. With the use of advanced techniques, surgery is becoming a more effective means of helping athletes continue their careers. Both Joan Benoit (Achilles tendon) and Mary Decker (anterior compartment syndrome in the shin area) returned from surgery to set world records. Arthroscopic techniques have made knee surgery much simpler. Instead of opening the knee to remove torn cartilage, the orthopedic surgeon can insert an arthroscope through small incisions and look for damage. He or she can then remove the damaged tissue if necessary. This method of surgery shortens recovery time from months to weeks.

Rest

Once regarded by doctors as a prime treatment, rest is now a bad word among runners. After all, how can you put zeros in your training diary! Few injuries require complete rest. Check with your doctor to find out what alternative exercise will be acceptable. However, you should rest until acute pain diminishes. For most minor cases of inflammation, such as shinsplints and Achilles tendinitis, a few days off the running trails combined with ice and aspirin will result in significant progress. Trying to run through inflammation usually prolongs the injury.

14 SPECIAL AIDS: INSOLES, HEEL LIFTS, TAPING, AND ORTHOTICS

Running is a relatively simple sport. The only equipment you really need is a good pair of running shoes. However, you may benefit from special aids placed in your shoes to help prevent or manage injuries. These include insoles, heel lifts, taping, and orthotics.

RUNNING SHOE INSOLES

Running shoes come with various types of insoles, which serve several purposes. They cover the inner shoe surface to prevent blisters; absorb moisture to prevent athlete's foot; absorb shock to prevent injuries and make it easier to continue training through impact-related injuries; and, in some cases, provide protection against overpronation. Insoles are usually removable and can be replaced, if necessary, by other devices, such as orthotics, or simply discarded if the runner feels uncomfortable with them. In most cases insoles should be removed if you wear custom-made orthotics because the insoles may interfere with proper functioning of the orthotic device. The insoles that come with most shoes are made of some type of plastic foam, which molds to the shape of your foot and provides some additional protection against overpronation. Check with your doctor or shoe salesperson for advice on which shoes have the type of insoles that may help you ward off or minimize injury.

REPLACEABLE INSOLES

Flat insoles are designed to absorb moisture, reduce the risk of blisters, and absorb shock. They are also used to adjust your shoe size if shoes are too big. They are not designed, as are orthotics, to support or control the foot. Insoles can be purchased at drugstores and running shops. Insertable insoles are simply put inside your shoes, either over or in place of the insoles that come with the shoes. They can usually be worn under orthotics to provide additional cushioning. Dr. Scholl's Pro Comfort Sports Cushions absorb shock well and are perforated to allow more air circulation. Spenco insoles are chemically treated to prevent blisters and calluses and also provide excellent cushioning.

Sorbothane insoles are used for maximum shock absorption. They are made from material that is claimed to be "similar in structure and function to human flesh." Sorbothane tests have shown their insole to absorb up to 94 percent of impact shock. Because these insoles are quite heavy (3 ounces each), you may choose to wear them only when warding off an impact-related injury. After you have fully recovered you can use lighter insoles, or Sorbothane heel pads, which don't weigh as much as full-length insoles but supply a good deal of cushioning. You might also wear full-length Sorbothane insoles only for distance training, especially long runs, and replace them with lighter insoles or remove them completely for speed work and races.

HEEL LIFTS AND HEEL CUPS

A heel lift is particularly helpful to a runner wishing to continue training while bothered by lower-leg injuries, such as shinsplints, Achilles tendinitis, and calf soreness. By raising the heel in the shoe, you are cutting down the strain on the Achilles tendon and the muscles in the lower leg, and thus minimizing the discomfort of your injury and helping prevent further strain. A "lift" of $1/4-3/4$ inches will help absorb shock and spread your weight over a greater area of the heel, thus combating heel bruises and spurs. Heel lifts or pads are manufactured by companies such as Dr. Scholl's, Spenco, and Sorbothane and can be purchased at drugstores. You can also fashion your own lifts out of surgical felt or powder puff pads. Build the lifts up to a height that gives relief, then gradually reduce the lifts until you no longer need them. Wear the lifts until a few days after an aggravation disappears. Make sure they aren't too high for your foot to fit properly in your shoe, and wear lifts in both shoes to avoid an injury resulting from imbalance. In some cases a runner may find it necessary to wear lifts all the time or to have them specially made by a podiatrist. This is particularly true in cases of unequal leg length. Simple heel lifts, when used at the first sign of a problem, often keep runners on the road and out of the doctor's office.

Heel cups are manufactured by several companies, including Tuli's and M.F. Athletic Company. These devices provide shock absorption, can help control movement of the heel, and distribute your weight over a greater surface, thereby relieving pain.

TAPING

The technique of taping, or strapping, has been used by athletic trainers in many sports for years. Its purpose is to allow an injured athlete to continue training and competing by providing support and control. It also reduces the possibility of reinjuring vulnerable areas. Taping may be used to help you overcome a minor problem or as an in-between measure while you are waiting for orthotics. You can be professionally taped by either your doctor or an athletic trainer, or you can learn to tape yourself.

Taping should follow these basic steps:
1. Shave all hair from the area being taped.
2. Wash the area thoroughly.
3. Spray tincture of benzoin compound on the skin to provide protection and help the tape stick.

4. Tape with 3-inch-wide Elastoplast (like an Ace bandage with adhesive) and 1½-inch adhesive tape for holding the corners of the Elastoplast.

Different taping techniques are suitable for different injuries. Dr. Weisenfeld uses four basic types of taping:

Arch Support Taping—for plantar fasciitis, heel spurs, fallen arches, posterior tibial shinsplints, or tendinitis (pain on inner side of leg)

1. Encircle the outside of the foot with tape. Attach the adhesive tape, starting behind the bone of the little toe, and pull it around to the back of the heel. Lay it on gently, applying no pressure. As you make the turn around the heel toward the inside of the foot, give the tape a little tug, so it's pulled tighter from the heel to the inside of the foot. Anchor the tape at the ball of the foot just behind the big toe. Smooth out any wrinkles in the tape.

2. Apply tape from side to side, along the bottom of the foot. Cut three pieces of Elastoplast, each about 4 inches long. Lay the first one along the sole of the foot, from just behind the little toe to just behind the big toe. Lay the second strip about three-quarters of the way over the first. Then overlap the third strip. When you're putting tape across the bottom of the foot, hold the bottom of the foot to keep it smooth. The skin should not wrinkle.

3. Encircle the outside of the foot with tape one more time. This is to anchor the entire strapping down and keep the edges from raveling. Use two strips of adhesive to tape down the edges and to anchor the entire taping down. Never wrap tape all the way around the top and bottom of your foot. This cuts off circulation.

You may wish to supplement the taping with a heel lift or a commercial orthotic to raise the arch and take pressure off the heel.

Taping for Pain in the Ball of the Foot. Pain in the ball of the foot is caused by bruised metatarsal heads, either on the bone attached to the big toe or under the second, third, or fourth toes. Taping a pad behind the metatarsal heads takes the pressure off the painful areas. Do not apply padding directly over the injury to cushion it, this will only further aggravate the problem. For taping:

1. Use a ¼-inch felt pad, sponge rubber, or a Dr. Scholl's heel pad.
2. Cut the pad in a U shape to fit around the metatarsal head. Find the spot by pressing your thumb into your foot until you feel sharp pain. Place the pad just behind that spot, in the direction of the heel.
3. Bevel the edges of the pad that point toward the arch.
4. Attach the pad with adhesive tape.

When you stand on the pad it should feel comfortable; if not, you haven't placed it properly. If you need more padding, glue another pad over the first one.

Taping to Control Supination. For mild peroneal pain and chronic ankle sprains.

1. Use 2-inch moleskin about 14 inches long.
2. Start under the inner anklebone and pass the moleskin under the heel, using no tension.
3. As you continue up the outside of the ankle and across the lower leg, apply tension. Be sure to pass the moleskin above the area of the ankle where flexion occurs; otherwise a blister will result. Secure the moleskin with nonelastic tape.

Taping to Control Pronation. For inner-knee pain, inner-ankle pain, posterior shinsplints, or tendinitis.

Use the same taping technique as that for controlling supination, but start under the outer anklebone. This will control pronation even in severe cases.

1. Use 2-inch moleskin about 14 inches long.
2. Start under the outer anklebone and pass the moleskin under the heel, using no tension.
3. As you continue up the inside of the ankle and across the lower leg, apply tension or the foot will be turned outward. Secure the moleskin with nonelastic tape.

PRESCRIPTION ORTHOTICS

Many runners have biomechanically weak feet. This means their feet have some basic flaw that, when aggravated by running, leads to foot, leg, knee, hip, or lower back injuries. With weak feet, the force exerted upon footstrike abnormally strains the supporting tendons, muscles, and fasciae of the foot and leg. Arch supports or orthotics often help runners with weak feet, leg-length discrepancies, and other biomechanical causes of injury.

Dr. Richard Schuster, a pioneer in the development of orthotics for runners, commented in *Running Review:* "The phrase 'orthotic foot device' is an impressive term that sometimes carries with it a bit of mystery. Actually, the synonym for the noun 'orthosis' is 'support,' so an orthotic foot device is one that supports the foot. There was a time when it was felt that the arch was the particular structure of the foot that needed support. Actually, there are several areas of the foot that could require support. The heel may require support against rolling the wrong way; the front of the foot may have to be supported in its natural position—which is not always parallel to the ground; and, of course, the arch may still require support. Also, orthotic foot devices for runners are designed to function in phases: heel contact, midstance, and pushoff."

Custom-fitted orthotics are something of a status symbol among runners nowadays. Many runners think of orthotics as a magic cure for all injuries, especially if their running friends all have them. If you think that you have a biomechanical imbalance or if you run over on your shoes but do not have pain or discomfort, leave well enough alone. Or, as Dr. Schuster advises those who insist on orthotics despite the fact that they have no real symptoms of injury, "Don't fix it if it works." Schuster warns that not all runners need orthotics: "Unless there are severe imbalances or pains related to imbalances, the indiscriminate use of orthotic foot devices could stir up a hornet's nest."

A survey of more than 1,500 runners at the 1980 New York Marathon revealed that 23 percent wore orthotics. This does not mean that 23 percent of all runners need orthotics, although many who increase their mileage up to 40–50 miles a week to train for marathons develop problems that can be helped with orthotics. Over 250,000 orthotic devices are prescribed each year for runners. We feel that 20 percent of these are not needed. Orthotics tend to be overprescribed because some runners who have been injured will try anything to get relief and often insist on them, and some doctors will try anything to satisfy their patients. By prescribing orthotics the doctor gives the patient something tangible to show for his or her money. But if the doctor doesn't find any imbalances, there is no reason to prescribe orthotics.

Orthotics can cause further injury through errors in prescription, construction, and use. According to Dr. Weisenfeld, orthotics are difficult to fit and mold, and thus errors do occasionally occur. Also, orthotics may impair runners' flexibility, their rearfoot correction is sometimes excessive, they need adjustment that runners don't bother to have done, and runners don't always break them in properly. Some runners can't tolerate orthotics.

A study by Dr. James Eggold, a California podiatrist, pointed out that 40 percent of 146 runners reported total relief from symptoms after treatment with orthotics; 74 percent reported nearly total relief. Other studies indicate that 75 to 90 percent of patients who are prescribed orthotics experience significant improvement.

Some runners who need orthotics resist them out of fear. Others resist them because of the cost: $150 to $350 including examination, lab fees, and follow-up examination. But if a competent sports doctor feels orthotics are necessary for you to run in comfort, don't resist. You may end up paying much more in medical expenses if your injuries get worse.

Here are the most common questions about custom-made orthotics:

How Do You Know If You Need Orthotics?

A major sign of your need for orthotics is the timing of symptom onset. If symptoms occur after a certain distance into a run, perhaps after 8 miles your knee starts to ache, or if symptoms occur after your mileage has reached a certain level, it is possible that you have gone beyond your body's ability to run pain-free with a biomechanical weakness. Another sign is if you feel more comfortable in a shoe with more support, or if you have some problems running on a particular slant. A leg-length discrepancy is another major reason for discussing orthotics with a sports doctor. If you are running fewer than 25 miles per week, you are not likely to need orthotics unless you have a severe biomechanical weakness that will not allow you to run in comfort. As your mileage increases, though, the strain on your body caused by structural imbalances becomes greater, and injuries are more likely to occur. Often a runner will get a series of nagging injuries one after the other; these are probably caused by a biomechanical flaw and can be corrected by orthotics. Runners who suffer from chronic knee pain, arch pain, plantar fasciitis, heel spurs, and certain types of muscle fatigue very often benefit from orthotics. If you have pain on the inside of the knee (chondromalacia or "runner's knee") there is a 90 percent chance that you can benefit from orthotics. According to a study of 400 runners by Chicago podiatrist Lowell Weill, 80 to 90 percent of chronic shinsplints sufferers need orthotics, and 75 percent can be cured by their wear. His study also reported a cure rate for heel injuries of 60 to 75 percent. But the majority of runners, even marathoners, do not need orthotics.

Where Do You Get Orthotics?

To obtain orthotics, consult a sports-medicine specialist who regularly treats runners and who is recommended to you by other runners. The first thing the doctor should do is take a history from you about your symptoms, weekly running mileage, running surface, shoe type, change in your program, and so forth. Then he or she will measure your range of motion, angular relationships, and possible leg-length discrepancy and perhaps take X rays. At this point the doctor can determine if you should use orthotics.

Taking a conservative approach, the doctor may recommend corrective exercises, perhaps a change in shoes and training surface, or commercial orthotics and taping. The goal is to manage the injury without having to burden you with the cost of custom-made orthotics. If the conservative approach does not work, custom-made orthotics can be prescribed. In some cases, where it is obvious that orthotics are necessary, the doctor will recommend that they be fabricated immediately. The runner's feet are then cast for orthotics and the impressions are sent to a laboratory for construction. Your doctor may decide to tape your foot so that you can continue running for the week or two it may take to get your orthotics.

After the doctor receives your orthotics, he or she should give you directions on their use, particularly on how to break them in properly. You may need to visit the doctor a few times to have adjustments made; the orthotics may be a bit too high in one place and cause blisters or need a little more lift under the heels. You will also need to have the orthotics adjusted to meet the demands of new symptoms that develop as you age and your training changes. The normal life of well-constructed soft orthotics is two to three years, depending on your mileage level and how well you take care of them. Hard orthotics should also last several years.

What Types of Orthotics Are Available?

There are two types of orthotics: hard, rigid devices and soft, malleable ones. Usually an individual doctor prescribes either hard or soft orthotics. Some podiatrists favor hard orthotics made of plastic or steel because they offer better rear-foot control and last longer. A flexible, semirigid orthotic offers some of the advantages of both hard and soft devices. Both these types of orthotics have some disadvantages for runners:

- Hard orthotics do not cover the entire bottom of the foot and thus provide less control of motion in the forefoot.
- Semirigid plastic devices are easily compressible, and thus may contribute to pronation. Rigid orthotics may not allow the heel to tilt properly. Runners with a limited range of motion usually have problems with rigid orthotics.
- Hard devices often aren't as comfortable; they have a rigid edge, which may dig into your foot. Most runners can accommodate a soft orthotic much more readily than a hard device.
- Hard orthotics must be sent back to the lab whenever a correction is made, whereas soft orthotics can be easily adjusted at the doctor's office.

Several types of soft orthotics are also available. The most commonly used is made from rubber butter, latex, and wood dust and is covered with leather. Devices made of rubberlike materials such as Neolite or Pelyte are a little softer than the rubber butter and may or may not be covered with leather. The softest orthotics are made of plastazote—a lightweight spongy material that compresses easily. These are used strictly for shock absorption and provide only minimal control. Some runners use these as substitutes for their full-support orthotics when they run speed workouts or races.

How Long Do You Wear Orthotics, and When Do You Need Them?

If you have a minor problem, you may use orthotics for a few months to correct it and then set them aside. Often, however, you will need them again if the biomechanical flaws that originally caused your problem are still present. You do not need to wear orthotics other than while running if you have only a minor imbalance or if you are not on your feet a lot during the day. For short races, 10 kilometers or less, you may choose to replace the orthotics with lightweight plastazote devices. But if you are a middle-of-the-pack or slower runner, you will be better served by having the full support of your orthotics. Only the faster runners who train in orthotics should consider not wearing them for marathons, but they should consider wearing at least the plastazote devices for cushioning and minimal control.

How Do You Break-in Orthotics?

Breaking-in orthotics too quickly can cause blisters and pains to muscles and joints that have been used in a slightly different way. Impatience in breaking them in or failing to see your doctor for adjustments can lead to further injury. According to Dr. Schuster, "one of the purposes of orthotic foot devices is to keep the runner running. However, there is a slight penalty to this in that problems that respond to orthotic treatment take a bit longer if the runner continues to run. A good rule—after the break-in period—is to run to the point where a suggestion of pain begins. If the orthotic devices are helping, one should be able to run increasing distances with comfort. Certain kinds of mechanical problems respond rather quickly; others take time. . . . As long as there are some continuing signs of improvement with the use of orthotics, the runner should be patient if he chooses to continue to run."

Here is Dr. Weisenfeld's recommended schedule for breaking-in orthotics:

Day 1. Wear them in your running shoes for 1 hour in the morning and 1 hour in the evening—for walking, not running.

Day 2. Wear them for 2 hours in the morning and 2 hours in the evening—for walking, not running.

Day 3. Wear them for 3 hours in the morning and 3 hours in the evening—for walking, not running.

Day 4. Wear them all day—for walking, not running. During the first four days you may continue running without orthotics if you can do so with minimal discomfort.

Day 5. Run 2–3 miles with the orthotics, then run the rest of your mileage without them.

Day 6. Run 4 miles with them.

Day 7. Run 5 miles with them.

For the second week, wear the orthotics for 1 more mile each day while running until you have adjusted to wearing them full-time. Do not wear the orthotics for runs of 15 or more miles until you have been running in them full-time for at least a week and have completed a run of at least 10 miles wearing them with no problems. If pain or severe discomfort arise during this period, call your doctor immediately.

COMMERCIAL ORTHOTICS

Over-the-counter, prefabricated commercial orthotics are made with semiflexible material, such as plastic or leather. They are contoured to the shape of the average foot and modified to reduce excessive pronation. Runners who suspect they need orthotics may use these devices before incurring the expense of custom-made orthotics. Commercial orthotics will help runners who have mild pronation problems or who run very little mileage. If your pain lessens but doesn't go away with commercial orthotics, or if symptoms return with an increase in mileage, then you should consult a sports podiatrist to see if you need custom-made orthotics. Commercial orthotics are sold in standard shoe sizes; the "one-size-fits-all" devices may produce good results for you if your foot size is close to the model used. Most runners, however, have differences in arch height, leg length, and range of motion that cannot be adequately corrected by such standard devices.

Some companies make inexpensive orthotics individually tailored to your needs from simple foot imprints and injury background information. We feel that if you need something other than over-the-counter orthotics, you could be headed for more serious injury by using these inexpensive but unprescribed devices.

THE RUNNER'S REPAIR KIT

Runners should be prepared to treat minor injuries promptly in order to keep in training. We have developed a runner's repair kit to help you in the self-treatment of injuries. Place the following items in a canvas bag or other container and keep it handy so that you can treat your injuries promptly:

1. *Aspirin.* To help relieve pain and combat inflammation.
2. *Heel lifts and insoles.* To give you increased shock absorption for impact-related injuries and relieve lower-leg pain.
3. *Emery board or pumice stone.* To smooth corns, calluses, and thickened nails before they become serious problems.
4. *Toenail clippers.* To clip your nails. Cut them straight across to minimize jammed nails or blisters under the nails.
5. *Ice packs.* In case you can't get ice when you need it, special ice packs that mix chemically to produce cold are a handy back-up.

6. *Moleskin or adhesive felt.* To make customized padding for various foot injuries requiring cushioning or support.
7. *Small scissors.* To cut tape, moleskin, and so on.
8. *Taping kit.*
   - Tincture of benzoin to spray on skin before applying tape
   - Elastoplast (elasticized adhesive tape)
   - One-inch adhesive tape for securing the edges of the elastoplast
   - Razor
9. *Blister prevention materials.*
   - Spenco insoles with chemically treated surface
   - Petroleum jelly
   - Talcum powder to sprinkle over feet and toes
   - Lamb's wool, Zonis tape, or Spenco Adhesive Knit to wrap toes and other areas that are prone to blisters
10. *Blister treatment materials.*
   - Gentian violet, Betadine solution, or other antiseptic to clean blister
   - Sterilized razor blades or needles
   - Gauze and adhesive tape
   - Spenco 2nd Skin, a hydrogel dressing that covers blisters and cushions the sensitive area to allow you to continue running

15 DRUGS AND RUNNING

Drugs are used by runners for three reasons: to improve athletic performance, to kill pain, and to reduce inflammation and swelling and promote healing.

DRUGS AND PERFORMANCE

Stimulants, such as amphetamines, may make an athlete feel as if he or she is performing better, but they have no effect on performance, can have harmful side effects, and may become addictive. Even caffeine, thought by some researchers to enhance athletic performance, was added to the long list of substances banned for use in the 1984 Olympic Games. The use of drugs, caffeine, or alcohol in an attempt to improve performance is fruitless as well as dangerous. If you've lost training time because of injury, don't panic and resort to chemicals in a desperate attempt to make up for lost time.

DRUGS AS PAINKILLERS

Dr. Weisenfeld cautioned in *The Runner's Repair Manual*: "Never take pain killers before going out to run, because they mask pain, and pain is a symptom. It's better for you to know that something's going wrong while it's happening. Otherwise, you'll keep running and with every step you're making the problem worse. In the end, it takes longer to heal and you've lost more running time than if you had stopped running when you first felt the pain."

Gary Muhrcke, a top marathoner for over twenty-five years and the first winner of the New York Marathon (1970), advised runners at a New York Road Runners Club clinic: "Don't be tempted to use something to mask pain so you can race. The Boston Marathon was very important to me one year, after I became a masters runner. I took something to block the pain during the race caused by a nagging injury. The result was that I was crippled as a runner for several months." Fortunately, Muhrcke came back from his injury and ran a personal record of 2:23:33, placing him only 14 seconds out of first place for age forty and over in the 1983 Boston Marathon.

Painkillers range in strength from aspirin, which reduces pain, but doesn't totally block it, to powerful oral drugs such as Darvon and injected drugs. The most powerful drugs recommended by your doctor should be used only while recovering from an injury, and not while running. Lesser-strength painkillers such as aspirin should be used after your run, but not for the few hours before running or during your run or race.

DRUGS AS ANTI-INFLAMMATORIES

Drugs such as aspirin, butazolidine, cortisone, dimethyl sulfoxide (DMSO), Motrin, and Naprosyn reduce inflammation and swelling and thus minimize pain and increase mobility in injured or overstressed tendons, joints, and cartilage.

Aspirin

In one form or another, aspirin has been around for many years. In 1893 a German chemist developed the standard aspirin tablet (acetylsalicylic acid); since then aspirin has become the world's most commonly used drug. According to Dr. Joan Ullyot in *Women's Sports*, aspirin is "not only very effective in reducing musculoskeletal pain, it is also the safest anti-inflammatory drug on the market, especially for heavy or prolonged use."

How to Use Aspirin. The standard aspirin tablet contains 325 milligrams of aspirin. Extra-strength varieties contain more, so be careful you don't take too much. Some products that are used as pain relievers, such as Tylenol and Datril, do not contain aspirin and thus do not reduce inflammation. The Food and Drug Administration warns that you should take no more than twelve standard tablets of aspirin daily and for no longer than ten consecutive days. Otherwise, you risk aspirin poisoning. Dr. Weisenfeld recommends taking two tablets with each meal and two at bedtime for two to seven days to help reduce inflammation. If aspirin causes you an allergic reaction or an upset stomach, use a buffered aspirin such as Ecotrin, which releases in the small intestine and doesn't cause stomach problems. Ascriptin is aspirin combined with Maalox; it coats your stomach to prevent upset.

Precautions for Aspirin Use. Aspirin can interfere with normal blood clotting, cause internal bleeding, and—if your stomach is sensitive—cause nausea and other gastrointestinal reactions. Because aspirin does not mask pain that is severe enough to cause further injury, some runners take it to help them train and race through nagging aches and pains. Some medical authorities, however, feel that aspirin should never be taken before running or racing because it interferes with the body's ability to warn you of further injury by sending out messages—pain. Aspirin also inhibits thirst while it increases the rate of sweat and the output of urine. Thus it is dangerous to take when running and racing in the heat because it can contribute to heat illness. Runners who take aspirin in heavy dosages and over a period of several days should be aware of the symptoms of aspirin poisoning: ringing in the ears, upset stomach, headache, dizziness, confusion, dim vision, sweating, thirst, and hyperventilation.

Butazolidine
Butazolidine is a powerful anti-inflammatory that is taken

orally in controlled dosages under the careful supervision of a doctor. It is so strong that it is used on horses, but it is banned for racehorses because it can successfully mask pain and allow a horse to race and risk serious injury. Butazolidine is commonly used to treat nagging inflammation in athletes. Bob Glover once used it successfully to clear up severe shinsplints that had him laid up for over two weeks. Your doctor should inform you that treatment with this drug is often accompanied by these side effects: upset stomach, nausea, diarrhea, and weight gain caused by water retention.

Cortisone

Cortisone is injected directly into the site of your injury. It is an effective anti-inflammatory and thus alleviates pain, but it should be used only when absolutely required. In some injuries an injection is the only cure for pain, because the injured structure lies very deep in the body and can't be reached any other way. Because it is injected locally, cortisone can be used in small dosages and affects only the area of the body where it is placed. Cortisone has a bad reputation because it has been used indiscriminately. Repeated injections into the same area can cause atrophy of muscle fiber and soft tissue and serious long-term injury. Used properly and conservatively however, it can be rapidly effective. Local injections can allow an athlete in pain to compete. In fact, some world record holders for the marathon have taken cortisone injections to compete in the New York Marathon. Remember, though, pain is a warning signal. The risk of further injury while running after receiving cortisone injections is great. If all else fails in your attempt to combat an injury and a competent doctor prescribes cortisone for *rehabilitation* purposes only, make certain that you receive only one or two treatments and that you are aware of the potential side effects.

Dimethyl Sulfoxide

Dimethyl sulfoxide (DMSO) is the most controversial drug of the 1980s. It is widely used and promoted by top athletes in every sport, including marathon world record holder Alberto Salazar. It is touted as an anti-inflammatory painkiller and miracle healing drug. But DMSO's healing claims have not yet been proven by scientific studies. The drug is illegal in some states, and cannot be prescribed because it has not been tested and approved by the Food and Drug Administration. The liquid is rapidly absorbed through the skin and into the bloodstream and may therefore carry impurities with it, resulting in still-undefined medical problems. Some athletes swab DMSO on after a hard workout or race to reduce swelling in injured areas. Others use it before a race to decrease pain. This is not recommended because it masks injury. Additionally, there are some unpleasant and potentially dangerous side effects: burning of the skin at the site of application, bad breath, body odor, bad taste in the mouth, burning on urination, light-headedness, and blurred vision.

CAUTION ON DRUGS

All drugs have the potential for uncomfortable, even dangerous, side effects. Generally, the stronger the drug, the higher the risk. If you need a drug to help you combat an injury, start with a mild over-the-counter drug such as aspirin. Your injury may eventually require a stronger drug, which your doctor will prescribe for oral use or inject locally. Oral drugs spread throughout your body via your bloodstream. Injectables, however, work at the site of your injury and thus can be administered in smaller dosages. Many sports-medicine authorities are not in favor of injecting runners, and most feel that injection should be used as a last resort for nagging injuries to the serious athlete. Remember, drugs may help you recover from your injury, but you must follow a sensible exercise rehabilitation program while you run through or come back from injury to eliminate or minimize the injury's causes. Don't become dependent on drugs to bail you out every time you overtrain. Do not take more than one drug at a time for any reason—such as medicine for a bad cold plus an anti-inflammatory—without consulting your doctor.

If your doctor prescribes drugs for your use in combating an injury, always ask three important questions:

1. Why is this drug being prescribed for me, and what are its benefits?
2. How exactly do I use it and for how long?
3. What are the potential side effects?

16 SPECIFIC TREATMENTS FOR COMMON RUNNING INJURIES

When a runner develops an injury, the specific treatment used should consider the symptoms, cause or causes of the injury, and rehabilitation. Almost all running injuries fit into one of the categories detailed in this chapter. Don't forget to review the questions to ask yourself when injured (pages 9–10) to help you and your doctor determine the cause of your injury. For a complete review of running injuries, consult Dr. Weisenfeld's *The Runner's Repair Manual.*

A runner should be treated for the symptoms of the injury as well as its causes, and a program of rehabilitation should be developed or the injury is likely to return again in one form or another. Bob Glover has had considerable success in helping his elite women runners return from serious injury through the use of alternative aerobic exercises and physical therapy.

Guidelines for coming back from a layoff caused by injury and running through injury are detailed in Chapters 4 and 5, and guidelines for using alternative aerobic training to keep in shape while returning from injury are detailed in Chapter 7. Chapter 17 includes some specific exercises to help with the prevention and rehabilitation of particular injuries.

A good example of how a coach can work with the medical community to treat and rehabilitate a runner with a specific injury is the case of Atalanta's Paula Morrell, who developed hip pain two weeks before the 1983 New York Marathon. She rested the injury and applied basic first aid—ice treatment. Because the race was important to her—she felt she could qualify in it for the Olympic trials—Paula started the marathon. For the first 18 miles she was running a great race on a cold, rainy day, but then her hip tightened dramatically, forcing her to drop out. She couldn't run for several weeks and felt pain even while walking.

Bob Glover asked Dr. Weisenfeld to screen her to determine which type of sports-medicine approach was appropriate, and, because he suspected structural damage, Dr. Weisenfeld suggested that Paula consult an orthopedist for a thorough evaluation. Dr. Fiske Warren diagnosed her as having iliotibial band syndrome, an inflammation of the lateral muscles connecting the hip and the knee, but no structural damage.

Paula then consulted a physical therapist for a rehabilitation program. It was discovered that she also had very inflexible leg muscles. Her treatment consisted of various physical therapy methods plus an extensive stretching and strengthening program for key muscle groups. Meanwhile, Glover designed a training program for Paula to follow: She replaced running minute for minute with swimming and biking and very gradually phased back into running. Initially, she also eased into speed work on the bike and in the pool before resuming speed work on the track and roads. She started with fewer repetitions and at a slower speed than she could handle if allowed to push; this enabled her musculoskeletal system to adapt gradually once again to the stresses of hard running. Less than three months from when she couldn't run a step, Paula placed second in a 10-kilometer race in Central Park.

KNEE INJURIES

Knee problems are a result of stresses and strains on the knee joint combined with the knee's inability to handle stress. Abnormal stress is caused by your foot striking the ground 5,000 times per hour with the force of three times your body weight when you are running. If something in the supporting structure gives, the result is often pain, or the inability to run.

The kneecap normally rides smoothly in a groove. It is attached to the large quadricep muscles of the thigh, which are strong enough to pull the kneecap sideways if the angle of the pull is twisted. The result may be irritated cartilage, which is symptomatic of "runner's knee," or chondromalacia. A variety of factors may cause this biomechanical problem.

Treatment Options for Runner's Knee (pain on either side of the knee)

Fight pain and inflammation by
- *Icing* the injured area immediately after the injury. Also ice it after all runs until the pain disappears.
- *Taking aspirin.* Stronger medication may be prescribed by your doctor if pain and swelling continue.
- *Resting.* Stay off the injured knee if it hurts to run.

Promote healing by treating the injury with ice, or using heat, massage, and electrical therapy for 48 hours after the injury to increase circulation and relax the surrounding muscles. Look for causes such as
- *Leg-length discrepancies.* Correct with heel lifts or orthotics.
- *Improper shoes or wear.* Check for improper support and sole wear, especially broken-down heel counters at the back of the shoe.
- *Slanted surfaces.* Avoid running on crowned roads, slanted indoor tracks, or beaches.
- *Overpronation.* Try taping or orthotics.
- *Muscle imbalance.* Strengthen the quadricep muscles; improve flexibility of the calf and hamstring muscles.

- *Overtraining*—too much mileage, speed work, or racing. Cut back until the injury improves; consider alternative training.
- *Incorrect form.* Watch out for overstriding, especially on downhills, leaning forward, and swinging arms across the body.

As a last resort, you can seek arthroscopic surgery. But be sure to consult at least two orthopedic surgeons who treat many athletes, including runners, before deciding on this remedy.

ACHILLES TENDINITIS

The Achilles tendon connects the powerful muscles in the back of the lower leg to the heel. An injury to this tendon can be painful and long-lasting. This is a basic inflammatory condition.

Treatment Options

Fight pain and inflammation by
- *Icing* the injured area immediately after the injury. Also ice it after all runs until the pain disappears.
- *Taking aspirin.* Stronger medication may be prescribed by your doctor if pain and swelling continue.
- *Resting.* This is a hard injury to run through unless it is quite minor. You may have to lay off anywhere from a few days to a few weeks. *Warning:* Continuing to train hard when you are bothered by this injury could result in a serious rupture of the tendon.
- *Not stretching* the tendon until the swelling and pain go away. Stretching will only aggravate the injury.
- *Elevating your heels* in your walking shoes and running shoes (if you are able to run with the injury, and when coming back from it) with heel lifts.

Promote healing by treating the injury with ice, or using heat after 48 hours, especially before bedtime. Gentle massage and electrical stimulation can also help the healing process.

Look for causes such as

- *Overpronation or supination.* Correct with taping or orthotics.
- *Overtraining*—sudden changes in mileage, speed work or hills. Cut back on mileage and eliminate speed work and hills until the injury improves; consider alternative training. Speed work and hills require you to push off hard from the toes, straining the Achilles tendon.
- *Poor flexibility.* After the injury heals, include special stretching exercises to improve flexibility of the calf and hamstring muscles.
- *Overstretching.* Beware of straining the Achilles tendon by pulling or jerking too hard.
- *Improper shoes or wear.* Check for wear in the heel counter, too much softness in the heel, or insufficient flexibility in the forefoot.
- *Incorrect form*—running too high on the toes, leaning forward. Run more erect, heel-ball, at least until the injury heals.
- *Soft or uneven running surfaces* (like the beach), which allow the heel to "sink in" or twist. Banked surfaces put more strain on the Achilles tendon than flat surfaces do.

As a last resort, surgery by an orthopedist can remove adhesions or sharp bone bumps that interfere with proper functioning of the tendons.

SHINSPLINTS

Abnormal strain and stress on the muscles and tendons that lift your forefoot and control your toes often result in shinsplints. These muscles and tendons absorb shock and stabilize your feet during foot plant. The angle at which the foot strikes the ground and the ability of the muscles and tendons to withstand the resulting force determine your susceptibility to shinsplints. There are two basic types of shinsplints: anterior tibial shinsplints, which involve pain in the lower front of the leg, and posterior shinsplints which involve pain along the inside of the lower leg and ankle. The causes of and treatment for shinsplints are similar to those for Achilles tendinitis, because both are lower-leg injuries.

Treatment Options

Fight pain and inflammation by
- *Icing* the injured area immediately after the injury. Also ice it after all runs until the pain disappears.
- *Taking aspirin.* Stronger medication may be prescribed by your doctor if pain and swelling continue.
- *Resting.* A minor case of shinsplints can be run through if you avoid hard training. Generally, if a runner suffering from shinsplints takes off a day or two the condition will clear up. Bob Glover once suffered from mild shinsplints but continued to train hard: He ended up not being able to run a step for two weeks. Continuing to push through shinsplints can also lead to serious stress fractures.
- *Elevating your heels* in your running shoes, or picking shoes with thicker heels. This will ease the pressure on the injured area.

Promote healing by treating with ice, or using heat or ultrasound after 48 hours, especially before bedtime.

Look for causes such as
- *Overtraining*—sudden changes in mileage, speed work, or hills. Cut back on mileage and eliminate speed work and hills until the injury improves; consider alternative training.
- *Muscle imbalance*—inflexible calf and hamstring muscles, which are relatively stronger than the quadricep muscles.

Do stretching exercises for the hamstring and calf muscles, strengthening exercises for the quads and the muscles that lift the foot.

- *Incorrect form*—running too high on the toes, overstriding, leaning forward. Run more erect, heel-ball, at least until the injury heals.
- *Improper shoes or wear.* Make sure shoes are flexible at the ball and have good cushioning and a thick heel. If shoes are too long or too wide, you may "dig" with your toes and cause shinsplints.
- *Changes in surface*—sudden switch from soft to hard surface.

For tenderness at inner side of the leg (posterior shinsplints) also check for these causes:

- *Leg-length discrepancies.* Correct with heel lifts or orthotics.
- *Slanted surfaces.* Avoid running on crowned roads, slanted tracks, or beaches.
- *Overpronation.* Try taping or orthotics.

As a last resort, surgery by an orthopedic surgeon may be required. Compartment syndrome is a "cousin" of shinsplints that is caused by abnormal pressure in one or more of the muscular compartments of the lower leg. It often requires surgery.

STRESS FRACTURES

A stress fracture is an internal shattering rather than a break in the bone. It usually occurs in one of the metatarsals in the ball of the foot, or in one of the lower-leg bones. The exact causes of stress fractures are not known, and sometimes a runner may even have one without being aware of it. If you can find a spot on the bone that hurts intensely when you press down on it, and there is a slight swelling at that point, you may have a stress fracture and should consult a doctor.

The fracture comes on slowly. At first it may seem to be a case of bad shinsplints, for example, but if the pain persists X rays should be taken. Sometimes, however, the fracture won't show up on an X ray for two weeks or so, and if the pain continues more X rays or a bone scan may be needed. In the meantime, treat the injury as a stress fracture.

Runners with poor footstrike resulting from improper running form or foot instability seem to be more vulnerable to stress fractures. So are runners who sharply increase their mileage or the intensity of their workouts. Even those who have never had problems and have followed a common-sense training program may suddenly find themselves with a stress fracture. This may happen because bone is a metabolically active tissue, and stress fractures can occur during a period of momentary weakness, such as jumping off a curb, running up a long hill, or doing a speed workout. Generally, it is felt that most stress fractures are caused by a bone not being able to withstand the increased stresses placed on it; when it fatigues, it develops the stress fracture as an abortive healing process.

Beware: Because stress fractures, unlike broken bones, are not always accompanied by severe pain and often seem like merely nagging inflammation, runners may continue running on stress fractures and end up with serious breaks. When in doubt, check with your doctor.

Treatment Options
- *Rest.* Rest is your only option. You must stay off a stress fracture and stop running for four to six weeks. Some doctors used to place runners in a cast to help the healing process, but most medical experts now agree that this is seldom necessary and could lead to muscle atrophy. In some cases, however, doctors feel it wise to put a cast on a stubborn runner to force him or her to stay off the running trails. Use

alternative training with a non-weight-bearing exercise, such as swimming or biking, to maintain fitness.
- *Orthotics* may be required to distribute weight better and prevent a stress fracture from recurring.

PAIN IN THE BALL OF THE FOOT

Pain in the ball of the foot may manifest itself in one of four ways:
1. Pain under the head of the first metatarsal, the big knobby bone behind the big toe, is usually caused by trauma; this is called sesamoiditis.
2. Pain under the second, third, and fourth metatarsal heads, those behind the respective toes, is called a stone bruise or just a painful bruised bone.
3. Neuroma in the metatarsal area, usually accompanied by a burning, stabbing, numbing sensation extending into one or more toes. This is usually caused by an impingement of a thickened nerve sheath.
4. Pain on the top of the forefoot over a very specific area, which is often a sign of a stress fracture of one or more metatarsal bones.

Treatment Options
Fight pain and inflammation by
- *Icing* the injured area immediately after the injury. Also, ice it after all runs until the pain disappears.
- *Taking aspirin.* Stronger medication may be prescribed by your doctor if pain and swelling continue.
- *Resting.* Stay off your feet for a few days if pain causes changes in your running form.

Promote healing by using *ice* or *ultrasound* for 48 hours after the injury.

Look for causes such as
- *Overtraining*—too much pounding with high mileage on

hard pavement, speed work, or hills. Cut back until the injury improves; consider alternative training.
- *Incorrect form*—running too high on the balls of the feet, leaning forward. Run more erect, heel-ball.
- *Improper shoes or wear.* Shoes that are too tight or too narrow will aggravate a neuroma; inadequate cushioning or flexibility under the ball causes pain.
- *Weak feet.* Custom-made orthotics will change weight distribution and relieve pain.

As a last resort, consider *surgery.* Removal of neuroma (soft tissue, not bone), is a relatively minor operation that can be performed by a podiatrist or an orthopedist.

PLANTAR FASCIITIS

Plantar fasciitis (arch pain) is an inflammation of the fibrous tissue that runs from the heel to the heads of the metatarsal bones in the ball of the foot. It is caused by irritation of this tissue, or fascia, and its separation from the heelbone. Plantar fasciitis is characterized by pain in the heel or arch when you get up in the morning and after sitting for long periods. You also experience pain at the start of your run, but it eases as you loosen up. Pushing off your toes to go up hills or to pick up speed aggravates this condition. It may be accompanied, but is not caused by, heel spurs.

Treatment Options
Fight pain and inflammation by
- *Icing* the injured area immediately after the injury. Also ice it after all runs until the pain disappears.
- *Taking aspirin.* Stronger medication may be prescribed by your doctor if pain and swelling continue.
- *Resting.* A few days off will help minor conditions, two to

six weeks off may be required to allow proper healing of severe cases. Consider alternative exercise.

- *Taking weight off the front of the heel* and *supporting the arch*. Heel pads or lifts take weight off the front of the heel. Taping or orthotics raise the arch, thus relieving strain.

Promote healing by using ice or ultrasound for 48 hours after the injury.

Look for causes such as

- *Overtraining*—too much mileage on hard pavement, speed work, or hills. Cut back until the injury improves; consider alternative training.
- *Improper shoes or wear*. Check for inadequate support in the heel counter, inadequate arch support, poor flexibility in the ball of the foot, or uneven wear in the heels.
- *Incorrect form*. Watch out for running too high on the balls of the feet.
- *Overpronation*. Correct with taping or orthotics.
- *Poor flexibility*. Do stretching exercises for the hamstrings and calf muscles.

HEEL BRUISES AND SPURS

Heel bruises are generally caused by stepping on sharp objects, such as rocks, or running too far back and too hard on the heels. They may simply require ice, aspirin, and a few days of not running to heal. Cushions under the heels will help you return to running sooner.

Heel spurs are very painful and the pain caused by them is long lasting. The pain is most severe on arising in the morning or after sitting for a protracted period of time and then arising.

Heel spurs are caused by the plantar fascia pulling very hard at its attachment at the heel over a period of time. Many of the microscopic fibers of the plantar fasciae tear away from their attachments and leave microscopic droplets of blood, which eventually form into a spur by calcification. The spur then irritates the soft tissue and a "bursal sac" is formed. When this sac fills with fluid and you try to stand on it, it hurts because the weight is forcing the fluid out. Heel spurs and bursitis usually cause stiffness and pain when you get up in the morning and may be painful at the beginning of a run, but they start to feel better as the run progresses.

Treatment Options
Fight pain and inflammation by
- *Icing* the injured area immediately after the injury, also ice after all runs until the pain disappears.
- *Taking aspirin.* Stronger medication may be prescribed by your doctor if pain and swelling continue.
- *Resting.* A few days off will help minor conditions, two to six weeks off may be required to allow proper healing of severe cases. Consider alternative exercise.
- *Padding the bottom of the heel* to help take stress off the area where the pain is. Place sponge padding in both shoes. This will relieve the pain by taking direct pressure off the area. Use heel cushion pads, 1/4-inch surgical felt, 3/4-inch sponge rubber, or plastic or rubber heel cups.
- *Redistributing weight* away from the heel with taping or commercial orthotics. Eventually you may need to see a podiatrist for custom-made orthotics. Dr. Weisenfeld finds orthotics to be the most successful treatment options for heel spurs.

Promote healing by using ice or ultrasound for 48 hours after injury.

Look for causes. Heel bruises and spurs have the same basic causes as plantar fasciitis.

As a last resort, a podiatrist or orthopedist can surgically remove excess bone or irritated bursa, or cut the fasciae away from the bone.

ANKLE SPRAINS

Ankle sprains can be caused by structural imbalance, improper shoes, rough terrain, and improper conditioning; however, they are most often caused by accidents while running, walking, or playing other sports. If an ankle sprain isn't properly treated, it can lead to chronic problems over the years. Ankle sprains result in torn ligaments, broken blood vessels, and inflammation, accompanied by pain and swelling. If you twist an ankle during a run or race, don't keep going in order to finish your run and worry about it after the run. It is crucial that you get off your feet immediately, even if you think it is a minor twist, and treat the injury. Swelling and damage happen quickly. If severe pain and swelling are present the next day, consult a doctor. He or she should X-ray your ankle to determine if you have broken any bones.

Treatment Options
Fight pain and inflammation by
- *Icing* the injured area immediately and applying compression and elevation. Continue icing for 48 hours.
- *Taking aspirin.* Stronger medication may be prescribed by your doctor if pain and swelling continue.
- *Resting.* Stay off the injured ankle until you can walk comfortably. Crutches may be used during the first 48 hours to decrease weight bearing on the injured ankle. Don't run until all pain and swelling have disappeared.
- *Taping* the injured ankle to provide support.

Promote healing by using ice, gentle massage, and gentle movement exercises. Consult your doctor for guidelines. After the injury has healed, and swelling and pain have gone
- Do strengthening and stretching exercises for the ankle.

- Do a few days of brisk walking before starting to run. Take a day off from running after any day that brings pain, swelling, or stiffness.
- Ice after each run until you have felt no pain or stiffness for several days.
- Tape the ankle before running for one to two weeks after the initial pain is gone.
- Run on smooth, even terrain, and avoid racing and running on turns until the injury is completely recovered.
- Make sure the outsides of your shoe heels are not overly worn.

As a last resort, your doctor may cast your ankle to provide support and keep you off it.

MUSCLE STRAIN

Muscle strains (of the hamstring, quadricep, calf, or groin) are a result of an actual tearing within the muscle group and are most often accompanied by inflammation. A muscle that is suddenly jerked by a sharp action or hasn't been properly warmed up will pull at its tendon or connection with the bone. Stretching exercises are essential for minimizing muscle strains. At the same time, runners can hurt themselves while stretching if they jerk hard and fast, or force a stretch. Strains come with bursts of speed, especially when the body isn't ready. Don't force yourself to push through tightness during speed workouts and races; warm up thoroughly first. Running on snow, ice, wet leaves, or uneven terrain will strain muscles. Other general causes of muscle strain include weak muscles (especially relative to opposing muscles), leg-length discrepancy, hill running, shoes with uneven wear or with inflexible or too-soft soles, running on slanted surfaces, overstriding, and running too high on the toes. If pain and swelling persist, you should see a doctor.

Treatment Options

Fight pain and inflammation by

- *Icing* the injured area immediately and applying compression and elevation.
- *Taking aspirin.* Stronger medication may be prescribed by your doctor if pain and swelling continue.
- *Resting.* Don't run until you can do so without favoring the injury.
- *Taping* or *orthotics* may be necessary to relieve immediate pain and chronic groin problems related to severe pronation.
- *Using heel lifts* will help reduce pain with hamstring, quadricep, and calf strains.
- *Running with a shortened stride* will reduce pain with hamstring strain.
- *Not stretching* injured muscles until all pain has disappeared.

Promote healing by using ice, mild limbering (not full stretching), gentle massage, and ultrasound to increase blood circulation.

BACK PAIN/SCIATICA

More than 80 percent of all Americans are victims of back pain at some time in their lives. With all the suffering, no one knows for certain what causes back pain. We do know, however, that overcoming most back pain can be merely a matter of flexibility and exercise. Low-back pain for runners is usually accompanied by muscle strains or spasms.

Sciatica is closely associated with back pain and is caused by the same problems. The sciatic nerve begins in the lower back and extends all the way down the leg to the ankle. Pain may occur in the back, the hip, the leg, or even the ankle and the two lesser toes. It may be a numbing sensation or a severe pain shooting from the back down the leg. Sciatica can linger for months, or suddenly appear and disappear, only to reappear again.

Severe cases of back pain and sciatica demand medical attention. If they are not treated properly, the result could be a chronic and disabling condition that might include herniated disk, degenerative disk, arthritis, or osteoporosis.*

Treatment Options
Fight pain and inflammation by
- *Icing* the injured area immediately and for the next 24–48 hours.
- *Taking aspirin.* Stronger medication may be prescribed by your doctor if pain continues. Muscle relaxants help relieve muscle spasms.
- *Resting.* Bed rest for a few days is often necessary in severe cases. Stop running until the pain has gone away, and then ease back.
- *Not stretching* the injured area until the pain has gone away.

Promote healing by treating with ice, or by using heat, massage, and electrical stimulation to increase blood circulation and relax tense muscles.

Look for causes such as
- *Weakness in key postural muscles.* If the muscles in the buttocks, the muscles along the spine, and the abdominals are weak relative to the hamstring, calf, and other "pushing" muscles used in running, back pain and sciatica can result. Do strengthening exercises.
- *Inflexible muscles.* Tightness in the hamstring and calf muscles causes a "pull" on the muscles in the back. Do stretching exercises.

---

* For more information consult *The Y's Way to a Healthy Back* by Alexander Melleby (Piscataway, NJ: New Century, 1982).

- *Poor posture.* Bad posture while walking, sitting, and running will strain the lower back.
- *Misalignment.* If your spine and joints get out of line, pain results. Manipulation can help you realign yourself and relieve the pressure on irritated nerves.
- *Improper shoes.* Shoes should have good cushioning to absorb the shock from pounding the roads and should not be worn down unevenly.
- *Stress and tension.* Back pain and tension go together. If you are going through a period of emotional stress, you may have to back off your running. Do relaxation exercises and avoid speed work and racing until your muscles are loose.
- *Leg-length discrepancy.* Correct with heel lifts or orthotics.
- *Slanted surfaces.* Avoid running on crowned roads or slanted indoor tracks.
- *Structural weaknesses.* Structurally weak feet and back may cause pain. Foot weaknesses can be treated with taping and orthotics. Curvatures of the spine cannot be corrected in most cases, but the supporting muscles can be strengthened by exercise.
- *Incorrect running form*—overstriding, especially on downhills; leaning too far forward or too far backward.
- *Overstretching*—forcing a stretch or bouncing. Don't do any stretches that tend to aggravate the back pain or sciatica.
- *Weight.* The more overweight you are, the greater the strain on your back.
- *Bad habits.* Learn to lift heavy objects (including your children) with your legs, not your back. Sleep on your side in the fetal position, not on your back or stomach. Sleep on a very firm mattress. Don't sit for long periods of time without taking a break to walk and stretch.
- *Overtraining*—too much mileage or speed work, too many hills. Back off until the condition improves.

As a last resort, surgery by an orthopedic surgeon may be necessary to remove ruptured or damaged disks. But try to treat the problem with corrective exercises first.

BLISTERS

Blisters are perhaps the most common and least respected injury the runner faces. If not properly treated, blisters can cause just as much trouble as any damage to muscles or joints. A blister is actually an accumulation of fluid under the top layer of skin, caused by rubbing. The area around the blister is sensitive to pressure, and redness and swelling are also present. The best way to deal with blisters is to prevent them: Eliminate the causes of friction. If you develop a blister during a run, stop immediately and treat it or you may lose several days because of infection. Running with a blister may also cause you to favor the injury and develop foot, leg, or hip problems. It is better to take a few days off and give the blister time to heal properly.

Treatment Options

Small blisters should not be punctured immediately. Keep the area clean and protected, and the skin may heal itself. Cover the blister with Spenco's 2d Skin or a similar product to protect it so you can run on it.

A blister that gets bigger and becomes painful to step on must be opened to relieve the pressure. Dr. Weisenfeld recommends the following procedure:

1. Sterilize a razor blade or scissors by boiling for 15 minutes.
2. Wash the blister with alcohol or an antiseptic.
3. Make a small slit in the blister and press the fluid out. Don't peel off the cap of the blister. Most of the pain will go away as soon as the fluid is released.
4. Clean the area with antiseptic. Gentian violet can be used to dry it. Ointment will not allow the blister to dry.

5. Cover the blister. Plastic bandages don't let air in, so use a square of gauze and tape it around the edges. Take it off at night to let the air at the injury. Use 2d Skin or a similar product to cover the area when running for several days after the injury to minimize further aggravation.
6. If redness and pain are present, you have an infected blister. See a doctor immediately.

Look for causes such as

- *Improper shoes.* Shoes that are too wide cause slippage; those that are too short or too tight rub.
- *Flaws in shoes or socks.*
- *Downhill running,* which causes the foot to slide forward in the shoe.
- *Friction.* Use Vaseline or talcum powder on your feet and in your shoes. Insoles such as Spenco also reduce friction and help prevent blisters.
- *Structural weaknesses or bumps* on your feet may also cause friction.

17 SPECIAL EXERCISES FOR SPECIFIC INJURIES

Exercises to stretch and strengthen key muscle groups are important in both the rehabilitation and prevention of injuries. The runner's cardiovascular system seldom breaks down, but the musculoskeletal system is vulnerable to a variety of injuries. Because running strengthens back muscles and those in the backs of the legs and makes them less flexible than the opposing, or antigravity muscles in front, a balanced program of stretching tight muscles and strengthening opposing muscles should be followed to minimize the possibility of injury.

Runners should use a regular routine of exercising key muscle groups. A proper warm-up and cool-down, consisting of relaxation, stretching, and easy running or walking, is essential. These routines help you prepare for and recover from each run and, if done properly, will maintain adequate flexibility and prevent injury. You may need to add more specialized exercises for particular strength and flexibility needs associated with specific injuries to which you are vulnerable.

The following guidelines for stretching and sample warm-up and cool-down routines are reprinted from *The Competitive Runner's Handbook*.

GUIDELINES FOR STRETCHING

The first requirement for increasing your flexibility is to learn how to relax. A few minutes of relaxing and limbering exercise release tension so that muscles can be stretched properly. Stretching exercises should condition the muscle and connecting tissues. A muscle works best when at its maximum length. Static stretching, which involves slow and rhythmic movements, stopping and holding at the point of first discomfort, should be done.

It is important to perform about 10–15 minutes of static stretching exercises before vigorous activity. The time you spend here will save time that would be lost to injury. At least 10 minutes of stretching and relaxation should be done after your workouts to prevent muscle tightness. The exercises are also of value performed during the day whenever you can, perhaps while you're on the phone. It all adds up to increased flexibility and a more fit body.

• Easy does it. Don't force it!

• Don't bounce or swing your body freely against a fixed joint—for instance, don't force a toe-touch with knees locked.

• Avoid overstretching. Too much is worse than too little. You can be injured by overstretching.

• Don't stretch injured muscles. Stick to easy limbering movements until the muscle is healed and ready to be stretched.

• Don't overdo stretching after a hard workout or race.

• Avoid exercises that aggravate a pre-existing condition—especially knee or back pain.

• Don't try advanced exercises too soon. Ease into each stretching routine just as you do with your running.

• Breathe properly. Do belly breathing while stretching, just as you do when running. Take a deep abdominal breath, and let it out slowly as you reach forward with your stretch.

• Warm the muscles. A muscle can be stretched safely only when it is relaxed and warm. Do relaxation exercises before starting. Some experts suggest that you run a few minutes first to warm up the muscles before stretching. We advise this before speed workouts and races, but not before your daily runs. Runners aren't likely to start their daily run and then after a mile stop to stretch. Start your daily run with easy relaxation and limbering exercises, and then some gentle stretches. Then stretch more thoroughly after you run.

• Include all major joint movements in your stretching.

• Include stretching for specific areas: hamstrings, calves, Achilles tendons. This is especially good when doing speed work.

• Older runners should work especially hard to stay flexible.

• Stretching in the morning, when you are stiff, can be a problem, especially the day after a hard race or workout. Try easy limbering and walking, followed by an easy run. A hot bath or shower first may help. Stretch more thoroughly upon returning.

• In cold weather, warm up thoroughly indoors, especially for speed work and races. A bath or shower might help, or an indoor stationary bike ride before your run.

• In warm weather, don't let feeling warm fool you into thinking you are warmed up and stretched. Be sure to stretch thoroughly.

• Don't be in a hurry. Take your time, and do the stretching step by step and thoroughly. Use the same basic routine every day so you feel comfortable with it; know it, and stay with it. You should never cut short your stretching just to get in an extra mile.

• Add to your stretching routine exercises for other parts of your body: sit-ups for your abdominals, push-ups for your arms and upper body. You may even add a few special exercises to your routine for specific strengthening or stretching: leg extensions for your quadriceps, for example, or additional stretches for your groin area.

Remember: When a muscle is jerked into extension, it tends to "fight back" and shorten. When the muscle is slowly stretched and held, it relaxes and lengthens. Reach easily and hold; do not tug and pull. The relaxed, lengthened muscle is more efficient, is less prone to injury, and recovers sooner from stress. Reach to the point of first discomfort, and hold for a count of ten. Then relax for a count of ten before repeating.

THE ROUTINES

Use the same basic exercises for your warm-up and cool-down, and the same exercises before each type of run you do. Here is a basic sample program to follow for all your runs. If you need to add a few specialized stretching exercises for specific problems refer to pages 189–196.

The basic exercises are the same for the three types of workouts—daily endurance runs, speed workouts, and races—although your total warm-up and cool-down routine will change to prepare you for faster running. Here is the sample warm-up and cool-down routine used for daily endurance runs, plus guidelines for adapting the routine to speed work and races.

The *warm-up* consists of three steps: relaxation exercises, stretching and strengthening exercises, and the cardiorespiratory build-up. You begin with relaxation to "break" muscle tension, which frequently causes muscular strain, especially back pain. These exercises also warm up muscles that are tense and difficult to stretch.

Here is a sample 15-minute warm-up routine. Lie on the floor with your knees bent. (You should always have your knees flexed when lying on your back, to relieve pressure on the lower back.) Do the following exercises in order:

Relaxation Exercises

1. *Belly Breathing.* Close your eyes. Take a deep breath, and concentrate on letting your stomach rise as you breathe in. Let go slowly and breathe out. Repeat two more times. To be certain you are breathing properly, place your hands on your stomach. They should rise as you inhale.

2. *Head Roll.* Same position. Roll your head slowly to one side, and let it relax there and go limp. Roll your head slowly back to the center, and then roll to the other side. Let go. Repeat three full rolls, right to left and left to right being one roll.

3. *Shoulder Shrug.* Same position. Relax, and as you take a deep breath, slide your shoulders up toward your ears and hold for a few seconds. Exhale, letting your shoulders drop limply to a relaxed position. Repeat two more times.

4. *Arm Limbering.* Same position. Raise your right arm 10 inches off the floor, make a tight fist for 10 seconds, then let your arm drop limply to the floor. Repeat with your left arm.

5. *Leg Limbering.* Same position. Slowly slide one leg forward until it is stretched flat on the floor, and let it go limp. Raise the leg 10 inches off the floor, and flex all the leg muscles for 10 seconds. Let the leg drop and relax, and slowly return it to the flexed position. Repeat with the opposite leg.

Lying-Down Stretches

1. *Double Knee Flex.* Same position. Pull both knees to your chest as far as you can without raising your hips. Then hug your knees with your arms, and bring your head to your knees. Let go, bring your arms back down to your sides. Lower your legs slowly to the flexed position with feet on floor. Repeat at least three times, up to as many as twenty.

2. *Double Knee Roll.* Same position—arms outstretched, palms down. Roll both knees together to one side until the outside knee touches the floor. At the same time, turn your head to the opposite direction and hold. Remain in this position for a few seconds. Then roll to the opposite side. Do one complete set three times.

3. *Lying Hamstring/Calf Stretch.* Same position. Bring one knee to your chest and slowly straighten the leg toward the ceiling, pointing the toe (hamstring stretch). Slowly lower the leg to the

floor and relax. Return to the flexed position. Alternate legs, and repeat for a total of two full sets. Then repeat the process, pointing the heel toward the ceiling (calf stretch), for a total of two full sets.

4. *Back Arch.* Same position, but with your feet as close to your buttocks as possible, heels on the floor. Grasp your heels with your hands, and as you take a deep breath, arch your back, lifting your bottom off the floor but keeping your heels flat and shoulders level. Hold; exhale as you return. Repeat twice.

5. *Cobra.* Lie on your stomach, arms at your side. Arch your back and look toward the ceiling. Hold, relax, and repeat.

Sitting Stretches

1. *Ankle Rolls.* Sit cross-legged. Grasp your right foot with both hands and rotate the ankle. Reverse direction. Repeat with your left ankle.

2. *Groin Stretch.* Same position. Place the soles of your feet together. Push down on your knees. Gently bend your head toward your feet. Hold the position with head down for a few seconds. Sit up; repeat two more times.

3. *Sitting Hamstring, Calf, and Back Stretch.* Sit with legs straight and spread, both hands overhead. Inhale, and then exhale slowly, and slide your arms along your left leg toward your left toe (keep the back of your knee flat against the floor). Reach as far as you can comfortably, and hold for a ten-count. Inhaling, bring your arms back overhead; sit up straight. Exhale as your arms reach toward your right toe, and hold at the point of first discomfort. Don't worry if you can't reach your toes. Repeat twice for each leg.

4. *Sitting Quadriceps Stretch.* Tuck your legs under you, sit on them, and lean back on your hands. Push your hips gently forward. Hold to a count of ten. Repeat two more times.

5. *Hip Stretcher.* Sit with your legs straight out. Bend your

left leg across the right and hug it with your arms, knee to chest. Hold; count ten; repeat with your other leg. Repeat twice with each leg.

Standing Stretches

1. *Total Body Stretch.* Stand with legs apart, arms extended toward the ceiling. Grab air with your right hand, then your left, alternating as you rise on your toes. Do this for 10 seconds, then let your upper body slowly bend forward at the hips, breathe out, and hang loosely as you slightly flex your knees. Slowly rise to a standing position as you inhale.

2. *Wall Push-ups.* Stand about 3 feet from a wall, tree, or lamppost. Place your hands on the wall, keeping your hips and back straight, heels firmly on the ground. Now slowly allow your straight body to lean close to the wall. Drop your forearms toward the wall so that you touch it with your hands and elbows. Keeping your back straight and heels flat, tuck your hips in toward the wall. Then straighten your arms and push your body back to the starting position. Repeat twice. Hold to a ten-count.

Next, stand close to the wall, feet together, hands on the wall. Bend at the knees, keeping your feet flat on the ground. (This is good for your Achilles tendon.) Hold for a ten-count. Repeat two more times.

3. *Standing Quadriceps Stretch.* Lean against the wall with your right hand. Reach behind you with your left hand and grasp the top of your right foot. Gently pull your heel toward your buttocks. Hold for a count of ten. Do twice with each leg.

4. *Upper-back and Hamstring Stretch.* Stand with your legs apart, hands clasped behind your back. Bend forward, bringing your arms overhead and tucking your chin in to your chest. Hold for 10 seconds. Slowly rise back to a standing position.

5. *Side Stretches.* Stand with legs apart, right hand on the side of your right leg, left hand overhead. Bend to the right at the

waist, also stretching your overhead arm to the right. Look up to the outstretched hand. Hold for 10 seconds, and alternate stretch to the other side. Repeat each side one more time.

Strengthening Exercises

1. *Push-ups.* Lie on the floor on your stomach. Then rise off the floor, back straight, so only your hands and toes touch. Form is important. Do five and work up to fifteen or so with good form. Back straight, fanny high, touch only your chest to the floor.

2. *Sit-ups.* Lie on your back, knees bent. Have someone hold your feet, or anchor them under a chair, bed, or bleacher. Put your hands behind your head, and roll up smoothly to a sitting position with your head close to your knees. Exhale slowly as you roll up and inhale while rolling down. Start with a few and work up to more. Do as many as you comfortably can with good form.

The Cardiorespiratory Warm-up

After the relaxation and stretching and strengthening exercises, begin a 5-minute brisk walk. Pick up your pace as you near the starting point of your run. Or start jogging slowly for 5 minutes, and then ease into your training pace. Don't go full throttle as soon as you begin your run. Allow your pulse to move up gradually and settle into your training range.

The *cool-down* is the warm-up in reverse: cardiorespiratory cool-down, stretching, relaxation exercises. It is also the easiest step to skip. But runners who miss their cool-down get injured because they haven't stretched and relaxed their muscles after a run.

After your workout, slowly walk for about 5 minutes. Follow this walk with the same stretching exercise routine as above, in reverse order, perhaps skipping a few stretches to make it a 10-minute routine. Don't do any push-ups or sit-ups. The purpose of the cool-down is to bring the body back to its pre-exercise level, ensuring the return of normal blood flow from the extremities to the heart and preventing muscle tightness. It is also important to slow your heart rate; your recovery pulse should be under 100 beats per minute at the conclusion of your cool-down. Take your pulse after your cool-down walk and stretch.

SPEEED WORKOUTS AND RACES

The Warm-up Routine

Before any fast runs, prepare your body for the stress. Bring your heart rate and breathing up to your aerobic exercise level, and prepare your muscles and joints for hard work. Your warm-up should include the following:

1. *Relaxation and Easy Stretching.* Loosen up. Follow the relaxation and lying-down stretches in the sample on pages 181–183.

2. *Warm-up Run.* Continue your pre–speed workout routine with a slow 10- to 30-minute jog before stretching further. For long races like the marathon, jog only about 5 minutes. This is a slow, leisurely, warming-up jog. The purpose is to loosen your body and warm it so that you can stretch more thoroughly. Some runners also find that easy runs of 2–4 miles in the morning before an early-afternoon speed workout, or a run at noon before an evening workout helps loosen them.

3. *Stretch.* Continue with the sitting and standing stretches in the sample.

4. *Pickups.* Run a set of six to twelve "pickups" or "strides" of about 60 yards on grass (if smooth) or on the road or track at increasing speeds. These should be brisk but not all-out. Do the first two or three slowly, concentrating on warming up your body and moving easily. Pick up the speed as you become loose; concentrate on good running form. This routine is specific dynamic stretching for the muscles and joints used in speed work and racing; it brings your heart and breathing up to the rates used during the hard work ahead.

5. *Relax and Limber Up.* Now do a 2–3 minute period of

light exercises, including head rolls, leg shakes, Achilles tendon and groin stretches, and any other relaxed stretching you may need. Do specific stretching for any area you feel is tight. Do not, however, perform these stretches in a nervous, haphazard manner. You are now ready for your speed workout or race.

6. *Ease into It.* If you are doing a continuous strength-training run, start at an easy pace to get your heart rate up into your training range and your muscles warmed before stepping on the gas. For intermittent track work or hills, run your first repetition conservatively, as a continuation of the warm-up. Jog into each start—never use a standing start.

For races, if the start is delayed after your carefully planned warm-up (begun 30 minutes before race time), keep moving, jogging easily and walking briskly. Avoid last-minute nervous stretching, which can be dangerous. Try to do a few more pickups right before the start, to bring your heart rate closer to race level. For the marathon, however, keep calm and try to conserve energy.

The Cool-down Routine

The cool-down routine is perhaps the most important—and often most neglected—part of your program. It helps you recover from your workout and be ready for the next day.

1. *Walk or Jog.* After your workout or race, walk around or jog easily to cool down. An easy jog of 1–4 miles will help you recover from the stress of the run. Next, walk around slowly for a few minutes until your heart rate returns to close to normal. Novices or those running marathons probably will be too tired to do any more running; they should walk. Do not sit or lie down. If you do, you'll tighten up.

2. *Stretch.* Follow your daily run routine. If your muscles are very tired and tight, do fewer stretches and don't force them. You may not be able to work your muscles as thoroughly, since they are fatigued. Be careful. Overstretching at this time can lead to injury.

Safety Note: If you do not have the time to do the whole series of exercises properly, select as many of them as you can do without rushing. It is better to do a few well than to do none at all or do all of them haphazardly. Here is a handy checklist:

SAMPLE 15-MINUTE
WARM-UP AND COOL-DOWN ROUTINES

Relaxation Exercises
1. Belly Breathing
2. Head Roll
3. Shoulder Shrug
4. Arm Limbering
5. Leg Limbering

Lying-down Stretches
1. Double Knee Flex
2. Double Knee Roll
3. Lying Hamstring/Calf Stretch
4. Back Arch
5. Cobra

Sitting Stretches
1. Ankle Rolls
2. Groin Stretch
3. Sitting Hamstring, Calf, and Back Stretch
4. Sitting Quadriceps Stretch
5. Hip Stretcher

Standing Stretches
1. Total Body Stretch
2. Wall Push-ups
3. Standing Quadriceps Stretch
4. Upper-back and Hamstring Stretch
5. Side Stretches

Strengthening
1. Push-ups
2. Sit-ups

Note: For cool-down, do the exercises in reverse order, from standing stretches to relaxation, ending with belly breathing. Then close your eyes and rest for 2 minutes.

3. *Relax.* End your routine with easy relaxation exercises. An easy swim, walk, or bike ride may help you recover from your workout—now, later in the evening, or the next morning. Afterward, of course, there is the runner's reward: the postworkout beer!

WEIGHT TRAINING

Proper weight training can help prevent injury resulting from imbalanced muscle groups and can strengthen your body for better performance. A regular strength training routine using free weights or weight-lifting apparatus, such as Nautilus or Universal, should be started, if possible, under the supervision of a professional instructor. For guidelines and a weight-training program, consult *The Competitive Runner's Handbook.*

Important muscles can be strengthened without the use of weights. Here are exercises to combat common injuries:

EXERCISES TO PREVENT RUNNER'S KNEE

Strengthening Exercises for the Quadricep Muscles

Do one or two of the following exercises on a regular basis. Weak quadricep muscles, or quads, can create an imbalance that affects the pull on the kneecap and causes pain. The solution is to strengthen these thigh and hip muscles.

• Sit in a chair, straighten your leg, and tighten it, holding the kneecap parallel to the floor. Tighten the muscles and hold for 2–3 seconds in isometric contraction. Repeat ten to twenty times.

• Sit in a chair with a 2½–5-pound ankle weight or metal weight boot attached. Straighten your leg slowly ten times. Rest, then do another set of ten lifts.

• Lie on a flat surface on your back with 3–4 towels rolled under one knee and a 2½-pound ankle weight wrapped around the ankle. With the knee in a slightly bent position, straighten the knee and hold for 2–3 seconds. Then lower the leg slowly. Repeat ten to twenty times.

• Hook your toes under a desk or couch and try to lift it with your toes. Your knees can be either bent or straight. Hold for 2–3 seconds. Relax. Repeat ten times.

• Stand with your back to the wall. Lift one leg as high as you can, keeping the knee straight. Hold for a five-count. Now bend the knee to relax for the count of five. Straighten the knee again. Repeat with each leg five times, increasing to the count of ten.

Do not do any deep knee squats or exercises lifting weights in which your knees are bent at an angle of 90 degrees or less.

In addition to these exercises, the following alternatives can also help develop the quads and prevent knee pain:
- Walk up several flights of stairs regularly.
- Hike or run up hills a few times each week.
- Walk in water, emphasizing the knee lift.
- Bike indoors or outdoors.

Stretching Exercises for the Hamstring Muscles

Tight hamstring muscles also pull on the kneecap. By increasing the flexibility of these muscles, you can minimize knee pain. The following exercises stretch the hamstring muscles:
- Lying hamstring/calf stretch (page 182)
- Sitting hamstring, calf, and back stretch (page 183)
- Upper-back and hamstring stretch (page 184)

These exercises may also be helpful:
- Place the ball of your foot on a table approximately 28 inches high; keep your other foot on the ground, with the toes pointing straight ahead. Bend the knee of the leg resting on the table as you move your hips forward. Hold the position for 30 seconds. Repeat twice with each leg.
- Place the back of your heel on a table, with the toes pointing toward the ceiling, and keep your other foot pointing straight ahead. Keep both knees straight. Slowly bend forward at the waist, looking straight ahead, until you feel a good stretch in the back of the leg. Hold for 10 seconds. Do three to five sets with each leg.

EXERCISES TO PREVENT ACHILLES TENDINITIS

Stretching exercises for the hamstring and calf muscles should be used regularly. *Do not* stretch the injured area until the swelling and pain have gone away. The following exercises are particularly helpful in preventing Achilles tendinitis (do one or two of them daily):

- Wall push-ups (see page 184).
- Squat down, keeping your heels flat on the floor. Your feet should be shoulder-width apart and pointed out slightly. Slowly bend forward and touch the floor with your fingers for support. Hold for 30 seconds.
- Sit on the floor, lean forward toward your outstretched feet, grasp your toes—if you can comfortably—don't force it—and pull them toward you slowly. (If you can't reach your toes, loop a towel around your feet and gently pull your toes toward you.) Keep your knees flat on the floor if possible. Hold for 10 seconds. Repeat five times.
- Place a slant board at an angle of about 15 to 20 degrees 8–12 inches from the wall. Stand on the board with your toes pointing "uphill." Lean toward the wall, resting on your forearms and keeping your knees straight. Keep your hips forward and heels down. Hold for 10 seconds and repeat. Repeat twice with knees slightly bent.

EXERCISES TO PREVENT SHINSPLINTS

Strengthening Exercises for the Quadricep Muscles

A muscle imbalance of weak quads and strong hamstrings and calves can contribute to shinsplints. See the exercises designed to strengthen quads and combat knee pain on page 190.

Strengthening Exercises for the Anterior Lower-leg Muscles

If these muscles, which lift the foot, are weak and the corresponding calf muscles are strong, shinsplints can occur. Use one or two of the following exercises regularly to prevent this problem.

• Sit on a table with your legs hanging freely over the sides. Flex your foot to lift a 2½-pound weight suspended from the ankle or foot. Do not lift the leg, just flex the foot and hold for 2–3 seconds. Relax and repeat for a set of 20. Then repeat with the other leg. To strengthen the muscles on the inside of the leg, repeat the exercise with your foot turned inward.

• Wall push-ups (page 184).

• Stand on the edge of a towel and curl your toes to pull the towel under your feet. Hold for 5 seconds. Repeat three times.

• Sit in a chair and put one foot on top of the other foot's toes. Pull upward with the lower foot as you push down with the upper. Hold for 2–3 seconds. Then switch feet. Repeat twenty times with each foot.

Stretching Exercises for the Hamstring and Calf Muscles, and Achilles Tendon

Use the same stretching exercises recommended for knee pain and Achilles tendinitis, especially wall push-ups (page 184).

EXERCISES TO PREVENT PLANTAR FASCIITIS AND HEEL SPURS

Strengthening Exercises for the Arch

• Do wall push-ups (see page 184) to stretch the fasciae.

• Stand on the edge of a towel and curl your toes to pull the towel under your feet. Hold for 5 seconds. Repeat three times.

Stretching Exercises for the Hamstring and Calf Muscles

Tight hamstrings and calves contribute to plantar fasciitis. Follow the stretching exercises for these muscle groups as recommended for knee pain and Achilles tendinitis (see pages 190–191).

EXERCISES TO PREVENT ANKLE SPRAINS

Exercises to strengthen and stretch the ankles will help prevent ankle sprains. These are particularly important for runners who suffer from chronic problems. Do one or two of these exercises regularly:

- Ankle rolls (see page 183).
- Sit in a chair; cross your right leg over your left. Rotate your foot in wide circles, clockwise and then counterclockwise. Do five to ten circles with each leg. Then, from the same starting position, flex your right ankle so your toes point upward. Hold for 2–3 seconds, then point the toes downward and hold for 2–3 seconds. Repeat five times, alternating flexing and pointing.
- Provide resistance by pushing with your hand against the foot in four directions—inward, outward, downward, and upward—and holding for 10 seconds. Repeat this three to five times in each direction.

EXERCISES TO PREVENT HAMSTRING STRAIN

Stretching Exercises for the Hamstring Muscles

After a hamstring injury has healed, improve flexibility by doing the stretching exercises for the hamstrings described on page 190.

Strengthening Exercises for the Hamstring Muscles

Do one or two of the following exercises on a regular basis:
- Lie on your stomach with a 2½-pound ankle weight on one leg. Bend the knee and raise the ankle to a 90° angle, then lower the leg slowly. Repeat ten to twenty times.
- Lie on your stomach with the backs of your heels about 2 inches below the base of a dresser. Lock your knees, and try to raise one leg up against the resistance of the dresser, pushing the back of the heel against it. Push up and hold for 2–3 seconds. Repeat ten times with each leg. Relax between each exercise.

• Lie on your stomach with your legs straight. Lift one leg as high as you can, keeping the knee straight. Repeat ten to twenty times with each leg. After adjusting to the exercise, attach a 2½-pound weight to your feet. Lift each foot up so the leg makes a 90-degree angle bent at the knee. Repeat ten times with each leg.

EXERCISES TO PREVENT QUADRICEPS STRAIN

Stretching Exercises for the Quadricep Muscles

Do the following exercises, as described in the warm-up routine in this chapter:
• Sitting quadriceps stretch (page 183).
• Standing quadriceps stretch (page 184).
• Lie on your right side with your body straight. Grasp the top of your left foot with your left hand and pull it back toward your buttocks so that the heel is as close as you can get it to the buttocks. Keep your ankle, knee, and hip in a straight line; do not raise the knee up in order to get your ankle to touch your buttocks. Hold for 30 seconds. Repeat two more times. Repeat exercise with the right foot.

Strengthening Exercises for the Quadricep Muscles

See the recommended exercises for strengthening the quads to minimize knee problems on page 189.

EXERCISES TO PREVENT GROIN STRAIN

Stretching Exercises for the Adductor Muscles
• Groin stretch (see page 183).
• Squats (see page 191).
• Stand with your feet spread slightly more than hip width. Your left leg should point forward and your right foot toward the side. Bend your right knee, and put your weight on your right foot. Hold 10 seconds. Now repeat with the other leg. Point the right foot forward and the left foot to-

ward the side. Bend your left knee, and put your weight on your left foot. Repeat five times.
- Sit on the floor with legs outstretched as far apart as possible and the backs of your knees flat on the floor. Slowly bend forward from the waist, trying to touch your head to the floor in front of you. Don't force it. Go as far as you can and hold for 5–10 seconds. Repeat three times.
- Sit in a chair with a large ball between your knees. Squeeze the ball for 5 seconds and relax. Repeat five times. Or sit on the floor with legs apart and place a chair between them. Squeeze the lower legs against the chair. Hold for 5–10 seconds and relax. Repeat five times.

Strengthening Exercise for Groin Pain
- Sitting in a chair with your knees spread apart, cross your arms so your hands are on the inside of the opposite knees. Slowly bring the knees together while resisting this movement with your hands. Repeat ten to twenty times.
- Do leg extensions (see pages 189–190) with toes pointed outward.
- Lie on your right side with your right hand supporting your head. Place your left hand on the floor in front of you for support. Your left foot should be flat on the floor in front of your right leg. Your right leg should be slightly ahead of your body. Now, flex your right foot so that the toe points up toward the knee. Keep the knee firm and straight throughout the exercise. Then lift the right leg as high as you can and lower it. Start with five to ten repetitions and work up to twenty. Each time you lower the leg, do not touch the floor with your foot and do not relax your leg. Keep it firm throughout the exercise. This can also be done with a 1-pound weight on your ankle. Turn on your left side, and repeat with your left leg.

EXERCISES TO PREVENT BACK PAIN/SCIATICA

Do the relaxation exercises to relieve tension on pages 181–182 and the stretching exercises for the hamstring and calf muscles in the sample warm-up routine (pages 186–188).

Stretching Exercises for the Back
Do two or three of these on a regular basis:
- Cobra (page 183).
- Kneel, resting on your hands and knees. Inhale, arch your back like a cat, tuck your head in chin to chest. Reverse: Bring your head up, exhale, and form a U with your spine. Repeat three times.
- Kneel, resting on your hands and knees. Slide both hands forward, bring your elbows and then your arms to the floor. Keep your back and head straight, your thighs perpendicular to the floor, hips up. Return to a kneeling position; rest. Repeat three times.
- Sit in a chair. Take a deep breath as you raise your arms up. Then exhale as you bend forward and let your arms hang between your legs, allowing your head to hang loosely from the neck.

Strengthening Exercises for the Abdominals and Postural Muscles
- Sit-ups (see page 185).
- The following exercises strengthen the abdominals, the buttocks, and the back muscles along your spine.
- Lie on your back, tilt your pelvis toward the floor, tighten your buttocks and stomach, and push the lower back into the floor. Hold. Count to ten. Relax. Repeat two times.
- Stand with your back against a wall, push your lower back toward the wall as you tighten your buttocks and stomach. Count to ten. Relax. Repeat twice.

INDEX

Abdominals, 69, 196
Acetylsalicylic acid, 154–55
Achilles tendinitis, 4, 6–7, 19, 22, 140
    exercises for prevention of, 190–91
    running with, 20
    treatment of, 162–63
Achilles Track Club, 86–87
Acupressure, 136
Acupuncturists, 125
Adductor muscles, 194–95
Aerobic endurance:
    biking for, 79
    cross-country skiing for, 111
    race walking for, 106
    swimming for, 90–91
    walking for, 102
Aerobic fitness, 70
Aerobics Program for Well-Being, The (Cooper), 111
Aerobic training, alternative, 67–78
    guidelines for, 72–74
    most effective, 90
    success stories of, 74–78
Aftermarathon, 51–64
    postrace program and, 53, 59–64
    prerace preparation and, 53, 54–56
    prevention of injuries in, 53–64
    race day preparation and, 53, 56–59
    See also Marathons
Age, running ability and, 5–6, 55
Alternative training, 46–47, 65–116
    biking, 79–89
    choosing of, 67–78
    cross-country skiing, 110–16
    race walking, 106–109
    swimming, 90–101
    walking, 102–105
Altshul, Victor, 30
American Academy of Podiatric Sports Medicine, 123
American College of Sports Medicine, 58, 123
American Heart Association, 102
American Massage and Therapy Association, 137
American Orthopaedic Society for Sports Medicine, 123
American Physical Therapy Association, 127
American Volksport Association, 102
Amphetamines, 153
Ankle rolls, 183
Ankles, 69
Ankle sprains, 171–72, 193
Anti-inflammatories, 154–57
Apophyses, 5
Arch support taping, 142

Arm limbering, 182
Arthroscopic techniques, 138
Ascriptin, 155
Aspirin, 154–55
Aspirin poisoning, 155
Avon Half-Marathon, 75, 76
Avon International Women's Marathon, 75

Back arch, 183
Back pain, 16, 173–76, 196
Backstroke, 97
Baths, hot, 60, 132
Beaches, 20
Beardsley, Dick, 103
Bell, John, 100–101
Belly breathing, 181
Benjamin, Ben, 129–30
Benoit, Joan, 49–50, 138
Biking, 46, 69, 79–89
　　benefits of, 79–81
　　guidelines for, 83–85
　　indoor vs. outdoor, 81–82
　　information on, 89
　　running vs., 82–83
　　sample training program for, 85
　　success stories of, 85–89
Blisters, 21, 152, 176–77
Block, Barry, 109
Boston Marathon, 20, 50, 58, 103, 116, 154
"Braking," 12, 20–21
Breaststroke, 97
Breathing, 81, 92
Brody, David, 99
Butazolidine, 155–56
Butterfly stroke, 97
Buttocks, 69

Caffeine, 153
Callen, Kenneth E., 29
Calories burned:
　　by biking, 79
　　by cross-country skiing, 111
　　by race walking, 106–107
　　by swimming, 91
　　by walking, 102
Chiropractors, 126
Chondromalacia (runner's knee), 5, 146, 161–62
Cleary, Mike, 83
Cobra stretch, 183
Cold treatments (cryotherapy), 129–31
Cold water, as cryotherapy, 131
Colt, Edward, 15, 61, 79
Common injuries, treatment of, 159–77
　　Achilles tendinitis, 162–63
　　ankle sprains, 171–72
　　back pain, 16, 173–76
　　foot pain, 167–68
　　heel spurs, 169–71
　　of knee, 160–62
　　muscle strain, 172–73
　　plantar fasciitis, 168–69
　　shinsplints, 163–65
　　stress fractures, 165–67
　　See also Treatment
Competitive Runner's Handbook, The (Glover and Schuder), 54n, 56, 92, 178–81, 189
Competitive running:
　　fitness and, xiii–xiv, 70
　　negative addiction in, 30
　　success in, xiv
Conditioning of Distance Running, The (Osler), 43
Coniff, James C. G., 124

Cool-down, 38, 185
    incorrect, as training error,
      13
    from speed work or races,
      187–88
Cooper, Kenneth, 79, 90, 111
Cortisone, 156
Costill, David, 40–41, 59, 61
Cross-country skiing, 46, 110–16
    benefits of, 111–13
    disadvantages of, 113–14
    guidelines for, 114–16
    information on, 116
    running vs., 114
Cryotherapy, 129–31

Daniels, Jack, 94
Darvon, 154
Datril, 155
Decker, Mary, 135, 138
Deep friction massage, 136
Deep massage, 136
Dehydration, 24, 57, 60–61
Depression, 30, 33
Detraining, 40–41
Diagnosis, from sports-medicine
    specialists, 124–25
Diathermy, 133–34
Diet, 16
Dimethyl sulfoxide (DMSO),
    157
Dirt trails, 19–20
Discomfort:
    pain vs., 24–25
    running through, 37
"Diseases of excellence," xv, 8
Distance, running:
    biking vs., 82
    cross-country vs., 114
    race walking vs., 108

    swimming vs., 95
    walking vs., 104
Distance runners, 38–39
Doctors. *See* Sports-medicine spe-
    cialists
Dr. Scholl's Pro Comfort Sports
    Cushions, 140
Dr. Sheehan on Running (Shee-
    han), 107
Doctor's Walking Book, The
    (Stutman), 104–105
Downhill running, 20–21, 177
Driving, 16
Drugs, 153–58
    as anti-inflammatories,
      154–57
    caution on, 157–58
    injectable vs. oral, 157
    as painkillers, 25, 37, 153–
      54
    performance and, 153

Ecotrin, 155
Edwards, Sally, 80, 84, 97
Eggold, James, 145
Eilenberg, Carl, 80
Electrical muscle stimulation,
    133
Ellis, Joe, 3, 4, 21, 121
Every Body's Fitness Book
    (Stewart), 90
Exercises, 178–96
    for Achilles tendinitis,
      190–91
    for hamstring, 182–83, 184,
      190, 192, 193–94
    for preventing ankle sprains,
      193
    for preventing back pain,
      196

Exercises (*cont.*)
　for preventing groin strain,
　　194–95
　for preventing plantar fas-
　　ciitis, 192
　for quadriceps, 189–90, 191,
　　194
　relaxation, 181–82
　for shinsplints, 191–92
　strengthening, 185, 193–94,
　　195, 196
　See also Stretching; *and spe-
　　cific exercises*

Fallen arches, taping for, 142
Feet:
　care for, 16
　pain in ball of, 143, 167–
　　68
　structurally weak, 15, 168,
　　175, 177
　taping pads to, 37–38
Flexibility, 163, 169, 174
　biking for, 80
　cross-country skiing for, 112
　race walking for, 107
　recovery rate and, 55
　stretching for improvement
　　of, 13, 38
　swimming for, 91
　of women, 4
Flotation devices, 94, 98–99
"Fluid loading," 58
Fluids:
　in postrace recovery, 60–61
　on prerace day, 56
　on race day, 58–59
Food:
　in postrace recovery, 61–62
　on prerace day, 56

Food and Drug Administration
　(FDA), 155
Footstrike, 13
　force of, 15
Form. *See* Running form
Fractures, stress, 5, 6, 19, 165–67
Frederick, E. C., 10
Freestyle, 97

Girard, Cindi, 88–89
Glasser, William, 29
Glover, Bob, 3, 12, 47, 53, 58,
　86, 87, 88, 100, 156, 159–60
Glycogen stores, 61
Goldstein, Seymour "Mac," 126
Greed, as training error, 4, 11
Groin strain, exercises for preven-
　tion of, 194–95
Groin stretch, 183
Gutin, Robert, 106

Hamstring/calf stretches, 182–83,
　184, 190, 192, 193
Hamstring strain, 193–94
Hard work recovery:
　biking for, 80
　swimming for, 92
　walking for, 103
Head roll, 182
Healing:
　gentle exercise and, 34
　psychology of, 32–33
Hearn, Angella, 47–48, 99–100
Hearn, Chris, 47, 48
Heart rate, alternative training
　and, 72–74
Heating pads, 133
Heat lamps, 133
Heat treatments (thermotherapy),
　131–33

Heel cups, 140–41
Heel lifts, 37, 140–41, 151
Heels, separation of bones in, 5–6
Heel spurs, 6, 169–71
    taping for, 142
    treatment of, 170–71
Helium-neon cold laser, 134
Henderson, John, 34, 62
Higdon, Hal, 93, 94
Hill work, as training error, 11, 37
Hips, 4–5, 69
Hip stretch, 183–84
Hoffman, Marshall, 119
Hot towels, 133
Hot water bottles, 133
Houston, Michael, 94
Hydrocollater packs, 132–33

Ice massages, 131
Ice packs, 130–31, 151
Ice towels, 131
Illness, comebacks from, 42–43
Indoor running, 20
Injuries, 3–25
    aging and, 5
    change in types of, 6–7
    comebacks from, 40–50
    environmental influences and, 8, 10, 19–23, 57–58
    of excellence, xv, 8
    four causes of, 8–23
    improper health practices and, 8, 9–10, 15–19
    from inactivity, xiv–xv
    inherited physical weakness and, 8, 15
    mileage and, xiii, xv, 3, 6, 10–11
    other sports and, 16–17

prerace, 54–55
psychological aspects of, 29–33
running with, 34–39
training errors and, 8, 9, 10–14
warning signs of, 8, 23–25
of women, 4
See also Common injuries, treatment of; Management of injury; Prevention of injuries; Rehabilitation
Injury and illness checklist, 9–10
Insoles:
    replaceable, 140
    running shoe, 139

Jackson, Douglas, xiii, 6–7, 12
Jacobson, Howard, 107–108
James, Stan, 50
Johnson, Brooks, 93
Journal of Sports Medicine and Physical Fitness, 61

Katz, Jane, 90–91, 96
Kidneys, 58, 61
Kneecap, 161
Knee flex, 182
Knee roll, 182
Knees, 20, 160–62
    biking for, 79–80, 84
    increase in injuries to, 6
    runner's (chondromalacia), 5, 146, 161–62
    of women, 4–5
Kropf, Robert, 5, 12, 91, 121, 127
Kwiker, Lou, 87

Ladas, Robin, 74–75
Laser, 134

L'eggs Mini Marathon, 89
Legs:
    limbering of, 182
    lower, stress fractures in, 5
    of unequal length, 15, 146, 161, 165, 175
Listen to Your Pain (Benjamin), 129–30
London Marathon, 47, 48, 49, 99
Long-distance running:
    excess, xiii, xv, 3, 6, 10–11
    young athletes and, 5–6
    See also Aftermarathon; Marathons
Long Island Marathon, 58
Lower back, 69
Lynch, Jerry, 32
Lyons, Paula Mara, 135

McDonald, Vince, 83
McKenna, John, 18
Mailhot, Carl, 135
Management of injury, 117–96
    drugs and, 153–58
    special aids for, 139–52
    special exercises for, 178–96
    sports-medicine specialists and, 119–38
    See also Common injuries, treatment of; Treatment
Manipulation, 137, 175
Marathonitis, 14
Marathons:
    environmental conditions and, 57–58
    fluids in, 58–59
    pace in, 56
    racing shoes in, 22, 57
    running form in, 57
    undertraining vs. overtraining for, 54
    See also Aftermarathon; Long-distance running; *and specific marathons*
Massages, 131, 135–37
Matthews, Leslie S., 4
Melleby, Alexander, 174*n*
Metatarsal heads, taping of, 143
Micheli, Lyle, xiii, 11
Mileage, excess, xiii, xv, 3, 6, 10–11
Milvy, Paul, 61
Mirkin Gabe, 71, 119
Misalignment, 175
Morrell, Paula, 159–60
Muhrcke, Gary, 154
Muscle development, balance of:
    biking for, 79–80
    cross-country skiing for, 111–12
    race walking for, 107
    swimming for, 91
Muscle imbalance, 14, 161, 164–65
Muscle pulls, 4
Muscles:
    in healing process, 32
    massage and, 135–36
    postural, 196
    "pushing" vs. "pulling," 7
    shin, 79–80
    See also specific muscles
Muscle strain, 172–73
Myotherapy, 137

Negative addiction, 30
Neurotic disequilibrium, 30–31

New York Marathon, 3, 49, 54–55, 57, 75, 86–88, 100–101, 145, 154
New York Running News, 110
Nike Marathon, 49

O'Connell, Sally, 115–16
Olympics (1984), 50, 88
Orthopedists, 126
Orthotics, 11, 15, 38, 128
  commercial, 150–51
  custom-fitted, 144–45
  hard vs. soft, 148–49
  prescription, 144–50
  semirigid, 148
Osgood-Schlatters disease, 6
Osler, Tom, 43
Osteopaths, 126
Overpronation, 161, 163, 165, 169
Overstretching, 13–14, 163, 175
Overstriding, 13
Overtraining, xiv, 10–11, 24, 54, 162, 163, 164, 167–68, 169, 175

Pace, in marathons, 56
Pagliano, John, xiii, 6–7, 12
Pain, 24–25
  degrees of, 34–36
  discomfort vs., 24–25
  distance runners' tolerance for, 38–39
  running through, 36–37
Painkillers, 25, 37, 153–54
"Panic breathing," 92
Parmalee, Patty Lee, 92
Physiatrists, 127
Physical therapists, 127
Physical Therapy Association, 123

Physician and Sportsmedicine, The (Ryan), 122
Plantar fasciitis, 6, 168–69
  exercises for prevention of, 192
  taping for, 142
  treatment of, 168–69
Podiatrists, 128
Pollack, Michael, 102
Positive Addiction (Glasser), 29
Positive thinking, 31, 32
Postrace recovery, 53, 59–64
Postural muscles, 196
Posture, 175
Prerace preparation, 53, 54–56
Prescription orthotics, 144–50
  breaking-in of, 149–50
  cost of, 146
  custom-fitted, 144–45
  need for, 146–47, 149
  obtaining of, 147–48
  types of, 148–49
President's Council on Physical Fitness and Sports, 102
"Pressure points," 136
Prevention of injuries, 8–25
  in aftermarathon, 53–64
  alternative training for, 69–70
  exercises for, 189–96
  orthotics and, 11, 15
  pain as warning in, 24
  running form for, 13
  special aids for, 139–52
  stretching exercises and, 6, 178–96
  swimming and, 94
Pronation, taping for, 143–44
Psychological problems, 29–33
  guidelines for, 31–32

Psychological problems (*cont.*)
    healing process and, 32–33
    stages in, 30–31
Psychosomatics, 29
Pulse rate, increase in, 23–24
"Pushing" vs. "pulling" muscles, 7
Push-ups, 185
    wall, 184

Quadriceps, 69, 79–80
    downhill running and, 20
    exercises for, 189–90, 191,
      194
Quadricep stretches, 183, 184

Race day preparation, 53, 56–59
Races, warm-up and cool-down
    for, 186–88
Race walking, 46, 106–109
    defined, 106, 109
    disadvantages of, 108
    guidelines for, 109
    information on, 109
    running vs., 108–109
Racewalk to Fitness (Jacobson),
    107–108
Racing shoes, 22, 57
Ratelle, Alex, 81
Recovery, 29–50
    alternative training for,
      46–47
    detraining and, 40–41
    guidelines for, 42–45
    inadequate, as training error,
      12
    planning of, 40–50
    postrace, 53, 59–64
    psychological, 29–33
    success stories of, 47–50
    time allowed for, 12, 41–42

    See also Alternative training;
      Hard work recovery
Reflexology, 136
Rehabilitation:
    biking for, 80
    cortisone for, 156
    cross-country skiing for, 112
    race walking for, 107
    swimming for, 91
    walking for, 102–103
    See also Alternative training;
      Common injuries, treat-
      ment of; Injuries; Manage-
      ment of injury; Prevention
      of injuries
Relapses, 12
Resting, 138
    conditioning and, 40–41
    running through injuries vs.,
      34
    after workout, 13
    during workout, 25
"RICE," 128
Road races, 19–20, 22–23
Roads, slant of, 19–20, 37, 161,
    163, 165
Rolfing, 136
Rowing, 77–78
Run Farther, Run Faster (Hen-
    derson), 34, 62
Runner, The, 4, 32, 40, 71, 81,
    93, 94, 124
Runners, old vs. young, 5–6
Runner's Handbook, The (Glover
    and Shepherd), xv
Runner's knee (chondromalacia),
    5, 146, 161–62
    exercises for prevention of,
      189–90
    treatment of, 161–62

Runner's repair kit, 151–52
Runner's Repair Manual, The (Weisenfeld), 153, 159
Runner's World, 6, 18, 84
Running, 30
Running & Fitness, 6, 109, 112–13, 135
Running diary, 25
"Running equivalent," 72
Running Foot Doctor, The (Subotnik), 42
Running form, 162, 163, 165, 168, 169, 175
    cross-country skiing and, 113
    downhill, 21
    errors in, 12–13
    in marathons, 57
    for prevention of injuries, 13
    race walking and, 107
    for speed, 13
Running Free (Ullyot), 110
Running Review, 144
Running through injuries, 34–39
    degrees of pain and, 34–36
    guidelines for, 36–38
    resting vs., 34
Ryan, Allan J., 122
Ryan, Eric, 75–76

St. Elizabeth's Hospital (Boston) Sports Medicine Runner's Clinic, 6
Salazar, Alberto, 48–49, 103, 135, 157
Schafer, Walt, 18
Schuder, Pete, 92
Schuster, Richard, 4, 21, 128, 144–45, 149
Sciatica, 16, 173–76, 196

Scientific Approach to Distance Running, A (Costill), 59
2d Skin, 38
Selye, Hans, 10, 17
Semple, Jock, 135
Sheehan, George, 23, 107
Shiatsu, 136
Shin muscles, anterior, 79–80
Shins, 5, 69
Shinsplints, 6–7, 19, 22, 140
    exercises for prevention of, 191–92
    posterior tibial, 142
    treatment of, 164–65
Shoes, 21–23, 37
    biking, 84
    flexibility of, 22
    heel counter of, 22
    improper, 161, 163, 165, 168, 169, 175, 177
    for marathon, 57
    purchase of, 22, 23
    racing, 22
    soft-soled, 6
Shoulder shrug, 182
Side stretch, 184–85
Sidestroke, 97
Sit-ups, 185
Skiing, cross-country. *See* Cross-country skiing
Slanted surfaces, 19–20, 37, 161, 163, 165
Sleeping, 16, 18–19
Smith, Lloyd S., 6
Sorbothane insoles, 140
Special aids:
    heel lifts and cups, 140–41
    insoles, 139–40
    orthotics, 144–51
    taping, 141–44

Speed, running:
　biking vs., 82
　cross-country skiing vs., 114
　form and, 13
　race walking vs., 108
　swimming vs., 95
　walking vs., 103–104
Speed work:
　anaerobic, 97
　swimming for, 48, 97–98, 100
　as training error, 11, 37
　warm-up and cool-down for, 186–88
Spenco insoles, 140
Spikes, 22–23
Sportsmedicine Book, The (Mirkin and Hoffman), 119–20
Sports-medicine clinics, 121–22
Sports-medicine specialists, 119–38
　choosing of, 123–24
　diagnosis and treatment by, 124–25
　requirements for, 123
　traditional doctors vs., 120–21
　types of, 125–28
Squats, 191
Static stretching, 179
Stegen, Art, 110–11, 113
Stewart, Gordon, 90
Stress, 17–18, 175
Stress fractures:
　in lower leg, 5, 6, 19
　treatment of, 166–67
Stress of Life, The (Selye), 17
Stress Without Distress (Selye), 17

Stretching, 6
　guidelines for, 178–81
　for improving flexibility, 13, 38
　lying-down, 182–83
　over-, 13–14, 163, 175
　routines, 181–86
　sitting, 183–84
　standing, 184–85
　static, 179
Stutman, Fred, 104
Subotnik, Steve, 42
Supination, 143, 163
Surfaces, 19–21
　changes of, 19, 165
　soft, 37, 163
Surgery, 138
Swimming, 46, 90–101
　benefits of, 90–93
　disadvantages of, 93–95
　guidelines for, 96–99
　information on, 101
　running vs., 95–96
　sample training program for, 99–100
　strokes, 96–97
　success stories of, 100–101
Swimming for Total Fitness (Katz), 90–91

Taping, 141–44
Tendinitis, Achilles. *See* Achilles tendinitis
Terrain, 19–21
Thorton, John, 61
"Tight" running, 12–13
Time, running:
　biking vs., 82–83
　cross-country skiing vs., 114
　race walking vs., 108

swimming vs., 95–96
walking vs., 104
Total body stretch, 184
Training:
    alternative. *See* Alternative
        training
    hard-easy method of, 12
    through injury. *See* Recovery
    for marathon, 54
    over-, xiv, 10–11, 24, 54,
        162, 163, 164, 167–68,
        169, 175
    shallow water, 99
Transcutaneous Electrical Nerve
    Stimulation (TENS), 134
Traum, Richard, 85–87
Treatment, 128–38
    cold (cryotherapy), 129–31
    electrotherapy, 133–34
    heat (thermotherapy),
        131–33
    manipulation, 137
    massage, 135–37
    surgery, 138
    trigger point injections,
        137
    See also Common injuries,
        treatment of
Trigger point injections, 137
"Trigger points," 137
Tylenol, 155
"Type-A behavior," 18

Ullyot, Joan, 110, 112, 128,
    154
Ultrasound, 134
Undertraining, xiv, 11, 54
Urine, checking of, 24, 60

Viren, Lasse, 135

Waitz, Grete, 49
Walking, 102–105
    benefits of, 102–103
    disadvantages of, 103
    guidelines for, 104–105
    information on, 105
    during recovery, 42, 44, 46
    running vs., 103–104
Wall push-ups, 184
Warm-up, 38
    biking, 80–81
    cardiorespiratory, 185–86
    for cross-country skiing,
        114
    incorrect, as training error,
        13
    for speed work or races,
        186–87
    three steps of, 181
    walking, 103
Warning signs checklist, 23–24
Warren, Fiske, 160
Weather, 19
    cross-country skiing and,
        112
    marathoning and, 57–58
Weight, 15–16
    racing, 55
    sudden loss of, 24
Weight training, 189
Weill, Lowell, 146–47
Weisenfeld, Murray, 3, 4, 5–7,
    53, 120, 124, 125, 142, 145,
    150, 153, 155, 159, 160, 176
Whirlpools, 132
"Who Do You Turn To?" (Con-
    iff), 124
Women, body structure of, 4–5
Women's Olympic Marathon
    Trials, 50

Women's Running (Ullyot), 128
Women's Sports (Ullyot), 154
Woodward, Bob, 112–13, 114

X rays, 166

Young, Kass, 76–77
Y's Way to a Healthy Back, The
  (Melleby), 174n

Zatopek, Emil, 101